Palliative and End of Life Care in Nursing

Sara Miller McCune founded SAGE Publishing in 1965 to support the dissemination of usable knowledge and educate a global community. SAGE publishes more than 1000 journals and over 800 new books each year, spanning a wide range of subject areas. Our growing selection of library products includes archives, data, case studies and video. SAGE remains majority owned by our founder and after her lifetime will become owned by a charitable trust that secures the company's continued independence.

Los Angeles | London | New Delhi | Singapore | Washington DC | Melbourne

2nd Edition

Palliative and End of Life Care in Nursing

Jane Nicol
Brian Nyatanga

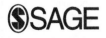

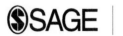

Learning Matters
An imprint of SAGE Publications Ltd
1 Oliver's Yard
55 City Road
London EC1Y 1SP

SAGE Publications Inc.
2455 Teller Road
Thousand Oaks, California 91320

SAGE Publications India Pvt Ltd
B 1/I 1 Mohan Cooperative Industrial Area
Mathura Road
New Delhi 110 044

SAGE Publications Asia-Pacific Pte Ltd
3 Church Street
#10-04 Samsung Hub
Singapore 049483

© Jane Nicol and Brian Nyatanga 2017

First published 2014
Second edition 2017

Editor: Alex Clabburn
Development editor: Richenda Milton-Daws
Production controller: Chris Marke
Project management: Swales & Willis Ltd, Exeter, Devon
Marketing manager: Tamara Navaratnam
Cover design: Wendy Scott
Typeset by: C&M Digitals (P) Ltd, Chennai, India
Printed by CPI Group (UK) Ltd, Croydon, CR0 4YY

Library of Congress Control Number: 2017936980

British Library Cataloguing in Publication data

A catalogue record for this book is available from the British Library

ISBN 978-1-4739-5727-5
ISBN 978-1-4739-5728-2 (pbk)

At SAGE we take sustainability seriously. Most of our products are printed in the UK using FSC papers and boards. When we print overseas we ensure sustainable papers are used as measured by the PREPS grading system. We undertake an annual audit to monitor our sustainability.

Contents

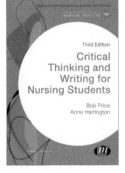

Third Edition
Critical Thinking and Writing for Nursing Students
Bob Price
Anne Harrington

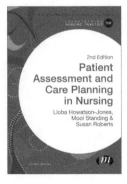

2nd Edition
Patient Assessment and Care Planning in Nursing
Lioba Howatson-Jones, Mooi Standing & Susan Roberts

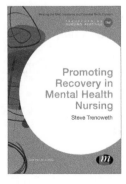

Promoting Recovery in Mental Health Nursing
Steve Trenoweth

CORE KNOWLEDGE TITLES:

Becoming a Registered Nurse: Making the Transition to Practice

Communication and Interpersonal Skills in Nursing (3rd Ed)

Contexts of Contemporary Nursing (2nd Ed)

Getting into Nursing (2nd Ed)

Health Promotion and Public Health for Nursing Students (3rd Ed)

Introduction to Medicines Management in Nursing

Law and Professional Issues in Nursing (4th Ed)

Leadership, Management and Team Working in Nursing (2nd Ed)

Learning Skills for Nursing Students

Medicines Management in Children's Nursing

Microbiology and Infection Prevention and Control for Nursing Students

Nursing and Collaborative Practice (2nd Ed)

Nursing and Mental Health Care

Nursing in Partnership with Patients and Carers

Palliative and End of Life Care in Nursing

Passing Calculations Tests for Nursing Students (3rd Ed)

Pathophysiology and Pharmacology for Nursing Students

Patient Assessment and Care Planning in Nursing (2nd Ed)

Patient Safety and Managing Risk in Nursing

Psychology and Sociology in Nursing (2nd Ed)

Successful Practice Learning for Nursing Students (2nd Ed)

Understanding Ethics for Nursing Students (2nd Ed)

Understanding Psychology for Nursing Students

Using Health Policy in Nursing Practice

What is Nursing? Exploring Theory and Practice (3rd Ed)

PERSONAL AND PROFESSIONAL LEARNING SKILLS TITLES:

Clinical Judgement and Decision Making for Nursing Students (3rd Ed)

Critical Thinking and Writing for Nursing Students (3rd Ed)

Evidence-based Practice in Nursing (3rd Ed)

Information Skills for Nursing Students

Reflective Practice in Nursing (3rd Ed)

Succeeding in Essays, Exams and OSCEs for Nursing Students

Succeeding in Literature Reviews and Research Project Plans for Nursing Students (3rd Ed)

Successful Professional Portfolios for Nursing Students (2nd Ed)

Understanding Research for Nursing Students (3rd Ed)

MENTAL HEALTH NURSING TITLES:

Assessment and Decision Making in Mental Health Nursing

Critical Thinking and Reflection for Mental Health Nursing Students

Engagement and Therapeutic Communication in Mental Health Nursing

Medicines Management in Mental Health Nursing (2nd Ed)

Mental Health Law in Nursing

Physical Healthcare and Promotion in Mental Health Nursing

Promoting Recovery in Mental Health Nursing

Psychosocial Interventions in Mental Health Nursing

ADULT NURSING TITLES:

Acute and Critical Care in Adult Nursing (2nd Ed)

Caring for Older People in Nursing

Dementia Care in Nursing

Medicines Management in Adult Nursing

Nursing Adults with Long Term Conditions (2nd Ed)

Safeguarding Adults in Nursing Practice (2nd Ed)

You can find more information on each of these titles and our other learning resources at **www.sagepub.co.uk**. Many of these titles are also available in various e-book formats, please visit our website for more information.

About the authors

Editors

Jane Nicol is a Registered Nurse and Lecturer of Adult Health Nursing in the School of Nursing, College of Medical and Dental Sciences at the University of Birmingham. During her clinical career she has worked in secondary, primary and third sector organisations and has direct experience of providing palliative and end of life care to patients, families and carers. Jane teaches on the Nurse Programme, where her input focuses on palliative and end of life care and long term conditions. She was shortlisted for a Nursing Times Award in 2015 and a Student Nursing Times Award in 2016 for her involvement in a student focused palliative care learning experience that aimed to enhance student nurses' knowledge and skills in relation to specialist palliative and end of life care. Jane has previously written for the Learning Matters series on the management of adults with long term conditions.

Dr Brian Nyatanga is Senior Lecturer at the University of Worcester, Institute of Health and Society, and Academic Lead for The Centre for Palliative Care, which he set up in 2013 in partnership with a local hospice. After spending the early years of his career working clinically in palliative care, he now teaches and facilitates palliative and end of life care, leadership and research methods to both home and international students. Brian is interested in emotional issues that affect clinicians and ways to support them to prevent the burnout syndrome. Brian recognises that working in palliative care can be a real source of stress and death anxiety; therefore, more needs to be done to prevent these symptoms from developing among clinicians. He is well published, and enjoys sharing ideas at national and international conferences.

Contributors

Chris Clarke is a Registered Nurse and Senior Lecturer in Advanced Clinical Practice at the University of Worcester. She has worked clinically in a variety of positions within the acute sector, predominantly within the remit of critical care, where she has gained experience in caring for acutely ill patients and their families, where decisions have to be made regarding the withdrawal and withholding of life-sustaining treatment, and in supporting organ donation through end of life care. Chris now teaches on the MSc in Advanced Practice, teaching advanced adult health assessment skills to nurses, pharmacists and allied health care professionals.

Jean Fisher is Head of Education at St Michael's Hospice, Hereford. Jean trained as a general nurse in Salisbury, Wiltshire, qualifying in 1979. Following a passion for plastic surgery and burns nursing she worked as both a staff nurse and ward sister in this speciality, developing both clinical skills and a deep interest in personhood and the impact of life changes and the importance of whole person care. Concerned about the lack of knowledge and skills evident in relation to caring for the dying and bereaved, Jean's interest and enthusiasm for palliative care grew. She first became involved in palliative care in 1984, when she was appointed as a ward sister in a new hospice. Since then Jean has been immersed in palliative and end of life care. She now combines education and management with some clinical activities within her current role. Her key areas of expertise are linked to pain management, communication skills and the development of professionals' knowledge, skills and confidence across the holistic spectrum of palliative and end of life care.

Hazel Luckhurst is a Senior Lecturer at the Department of Nursing and Midwifery, University of Worcester. Her areas of expertise include critical care, leadership and problem-based learning. Hazel has extensive experience in critical care subspecialties such as cardiothoracic, trauma and general and neuroscience intensive care both in the UK and overseas. In addition, Hazel has direct bedside clinical experience supporting critically ill patients at the end of life. Hazel has led diploma and degree critical care modules and teaches across nursing programmes which address the dynamic nature of professional health care.

Sherri Ogston-Tuck is Senior Lecturer with the Department of Nursing and Midwifery, Institute of Health and Society at the University of Worcester. Her clinical background is in acute adult nursing with an emphasis in law and ethics, pain and medicines management. Sherri undertook her nurse education and training in Canada; she now has 20 years of clinical nursing experience in emergency and acute adult care in the UK. Sherri has worked in an academic role for over a decade and has a range of publications to her name. Sherri's interest in law and ethics in nursing practice has developed as a result of the emerging role and responsibilities of the nurse, the complexities of the human condition and decision making in health care today. Sherri's Chapter 6 is dedicated to Douglas Ogston who, in his end of life care, was given kindness and care by hospice staff and volunteers, and was not alone when he needed his family most.

Dr Helen Taylor is a Principal Lecturer at the Institute of Health and Society at the University of Worcester. She has a PhD in Health Psychology and is a barrister. Helen has a long-standing research and academic interest, together with a range of publications focusing on the promotion of an individual's right to autonomy, dignity and respect.

Acknowledgements

This second edition would not have been complete without new ideas and insight from the editorial team and support of the contributors. You will see that there are new ideas highlighting real challenges to delivering the best possible palliative care. I hope this edition will enhance current thinking and more importantly, you find it user-friendly. In a more general way, I would like to thank all contributors for giving up their precious time from their busy worlds to share their insights in this edition.

In a more special way, I would to make the following dedication:

To Priscilla, Pamela Lou, Nev, Lewin.

To my mother who died last year at the age of 105 years; I salute your greatness and sense of fairness always.

Brian Nyatanga

Introduction

About this book

The main aim of the book is to discuss some of the key aspects of palliative and end of life care in a way that aids understanding. This book is written and edited by experts in the field of palliative and end of life care, and offers the reader an introduction to one of the most complex and sensitive areas of health care practice. The book is written, in the main, for those entering health care professions like student nurses, student doctors and allied health professionals, who wish to develop their understanding in palliative and end of life care. It is also envisaged that more experienced health care professionals can use this book as a refresher and aide when teaching other members of staff.

Why palliative and end of life care?

The title of the book recognises the sometimes long journey from diagnosis to death which characterises palliative care and the end point/final phase of life before physical death (end of life). This can bring about complex emotions and reactions. Palliative and end of life cares requires a comprehensive supportive approach by health care professionals to ensure all those in need are helped, cared for and supported in order to adjust to impending death and beyond.

Book structure

The book comprises eight chapters, each focusing on an important aspect of palliative care. Although the book can be read by dipping in and out of chapters, it is recommended that Chapter 1 is read first as this sets the scene to some of the philosophical positions encountered in life, living, dying and death. It is suggested that appreciating some of this philosophical discourse is needed before fully understanding the delivery and practice of palliative and end of life care. Chapter 2 looks at the important and yet difficult aspect of communicating with a dying patient. A number of skills that facilitate effective communication are discussed while potential barriers are also highlighted. Communication is, in essence, the glue that binds everything we do in caring and should always be practised and perfected. Chapter 3 acknowledges that dying and death provoke a sense of loss which is followed by grief, both of which need to be managed through bereavement. This chapter uses some well-known theories and models of loss, grief and bereavement to help the reader to understand how patients and families may react to death and dying. Chapter 4 recognises the changing multi-cultural nature of the UK population and indeed most countries, and therefore discusses the ideas of culture, culture modifications and the need to be culturally competent to care for patients from different cultural backgrounds. Chapter 5 focuses on rehabilitation in palliative and end of life care. For people receiving palliative and end of life care rehabilitation can support them to 'live well', maximising their ability to maintain choice, control and independence. In this chapter the topic of living with and beyond cancer is introduced; rehabilitation plays a key role in supporting people to manage the long term consequences of their disease and treatment. Chapter 6 explores the core ethical principles in health care and relates these to particular palliative and end of life care scenarios. In doing this the chapter provides a framework for practice that can be used to inform practice when challenging decisions about treatment options are present. Given the close relationship between ethics and legal aspects of care readers are encouraged to read these chapters together. Chapter 7 discusses delivering palliative care in an intensive care unit, the shift in care this requires and some of the challenges present. This environment is rarely seen as palliative care and yet a number of people die here each year. By discussing palliative care in an intensive care unit, this chapter illustrates that the philosophy of palliative care can be practised anywhere as long as someone is dying. Chapter 8 is the final chapter for this book and gives a series of legal cases that happened in this country as a way of demonstrating the complexity of some of the deliberations lawyers and judges go through and the decisions they make. It is clear that there is a clear distinction between the legal and professional positions when caring for other people, and carers in palliative care need to be aware of these.

Standards for Pre-registration Nursing Education and Essential Skills Clusters

These standards (NMC, 2010) are used by those planning pre-registration nursing education courses. At the beginning of each chapter there is a guide to the most relevant domains and competencies described in the standards. However, this may not be exhaustive and readers should consult the full standards to support their own learning. The four domains, with their respective generic standards for competence, are as follows.

1. Domain 1: Professional values

    a. All nurses must act first and foremost to care for and safeguard the public. They must practise autonomously and be responsible and accountable for safe, compassionate, person-centred, evidence-based nursing care that respects and maintains dignity and human rights. They must show professionalism and integrity and work within recognised professional, ethical and legal frameworks. They must work in partnership with other health and social care professionals and agencies, service users, their carers and families in all settings, including the community, ensuring that decisions about care are shared.

2. Domain 2: Communication and interpersonal skills

    b. All nurses must use excellent communication and interpersonal skills. Their communications must always be safe, effective, compassionate and respectful. They must communicate effectively using a wide range of strategies and interventions including the effective use of communication technologies. Where people have a disability, nurses must be able to work with service users and others to obtain the information they need to make reasonable adjustments that promote optimum health and enable equal access to services.

3. Domain 3: Nursing practice and decision-making

    c. All nurses must practise autonomously, compassionately, skilfully and safely, and must maintain dignity and promote health and wellbeing. They must assess and meet the full range of essential physical and mental health needs of people of all ages who come into their care. Where necessary they must be able to provide safe and effective immediate care to all people prior to accessing or referring to specialist services irrespective of their field of practice. All nurses must be able to meet more complex and coexisting needs for people in their own nursing field of practice, in any setting including hospital, community and at home. All practice should be informed by the best available evidence and comply with local and national guidelines. Decision-making must be shared with service users, carers and families and informed by critical analysis of a full range of possible interventions, including the use of up-to-date technology. All nurses must also understand how behaviour, culture, socioeconomic and other factors, in the care environment and its location, can affect health, illness, health outcomes and public health priorities and take into account planning and delivering care.

4. Domain: Leadership, management and team working

    d. All nurses must be professionally accountable and use clinical governance processes to maintain and improve nursing practice and standards of health care. They must be able to respond autonomously and confidently to planned and uncertain situations, managing themselves and others effectively. They must create and maximise opportunities to improve service. They must also demonstrate the potential to develop further management and leadership skills during their period of preceptorship and beyond.

The NMC states that the Essential Skills Clusters (ESCs) must be part of all pre-registration nursing courses. How this is done is up to those who are planning how the course will be delivered. There are five skills clusters in total:

*   care, compassion and communication;
*   organisational aspects of care;
*   infection prevention and control;
*   nutrition and fluid management;
*   medicines management.

These ESCs are designed to support the achievement of the competencies listed under each of the four domains. Some chapters in this book are particularly relevant to certain clusters, and this will be highlighted as appropriate.

Learning features

Throughout the book you will find activities in the text that will help you to make sense of, and learn about, the material being presented by the authors.

Some activities ask you to *reflect* on aspects of practice, or your experience of it, or the people or situations you encounter. Other activities will help you develop key skills such as your ability to *think critically* about a topic in order to challenge received wisdom, or your ability to *research a topic and find appropriate information and evidence*, and to be able to make decisions using that evidence in situations that are often difficult and time-pressured. Finally, communication and working as part of a team are core to all nursing practice, and some activities will ask you to carry out *group activities* or think about your *communication skills* to help develop these.

All the activities require you to take a break from reading the text, think through the issues presented and carry out some independent study, possibly using the internet. Where appropriate, there are sample answers presented at the end of each chapter, and these will help you to understand more fully your own reflections and independent study.

Chapter 1
The idea of living, dying, life and death

Brian Nyatanga

NMC Standards for Pre-registration Nursing Education

This chapter will address the following competencies:

Domain 1: Professional values

2. All nurses must practise in a holistic, non-judgemental, caring and sensitive manner that avoids assumptions, supports social inclusion; recognises and respects individual choice; and acknowledges diversity. Where necessary, they must challenge inequality, discrimination and exclusion from access to care.

Domain 2: Communication and interpersonal skills

1. All nurses must build partnerships and therapeutic relationships through effective and non-discriminatory communication. They must take account of individual differences, capabilities and needs.

Domain 3: Nursing practice and decision-making

4. All nurses must ascertain and respond to the physical, social and psychological needs of people, groups and communities. They must then plan, deliver and evaluate safe, competent, person-centred care in partnership with them, paying special attention to changing health needs during different life stages, including progressive illness and death, loss and bereavement.

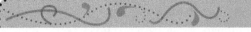

NMC Essential Skills Clusters

This chapter will address the following ESCs:

Cluster: care, compassion and communication

3. People can trust the newly registered graduate nurse to respect them as individuals and strive to help them preserve their dignity at all times.

continued … •

First progression point

1. Demonstrate respect for diversity and individual preference, valuing differences, regardless of personal view.

Entry to the register

4. Acts professionally to ensure that personal judgements, prejudices, values, attitudes and beliefs do not compromise care.

Chapter aims

After reading this chapter, you will be able to:

- understand the connection between living and dying, and then between life and death in the context of palliative care and end of life care;
- appreciate the possible reasons many people fear death, and how you can support patients to achieve a dignified death for them;
- appreciate the role euphemisms play in 'softening' the reality of death and the impact this can have on patients and the bereaved;
- understand what palliative and end of life care are and their underlying ethos;
- appreciate the importance of dying in your own home and use this information to support patient-centred palliative and end of life care.

Introduction

Si vis vitam para mortem
If you wish for life, prepare yourself for death

The key message of this saying is that although life and death may present differently, they are part of the same thing. The two realities are perceived as being on a continuum but positioned at two distinct polarities (ends) with life at the beginning and death at the other end. These two realities cannot be separated – we cannot experience one without the other – therefore we need to find a way of reconciling them. The truth is that human beings have no choice between these two realities although the popular belief is that life is always preferable to death. Therefore every effort is made to enjoy life while doing everything possible to delay death. In this paradox, we can also see deep seated conceptual denial of death and an overwhelming but often misplaced optimism about human immortality. Freud summed this up in his 1953 celebrated statement that death was unimaginable and therefore not available:

> *It is indeed impossible to imagine our own death; and whenever we attempt to do so we can perceive that we are still present as spectators.*

In other words, Freud was arguing that at our unconscious level we are all convinced that we are immortal. Looking at this closely we have to ask and wonder whether this is our way of coping with the threat of death and therefore a defence mechanism against the anxiety (death anxiety) that can be experienced.

The saying at the start also identifies some philosophical ideas about the interconnectedness of life and death – which can be experienced through living and which can be realised (reached) through the dying process. It is no secret that most people tend to fear death even though they all know it will happen to them at some point in their life.

The aim of this chapter is to allow you to explore this paradox, and similar conflicting ideas surrounding life and death, and to use this knowledge to enable you to provide person-centred care for patients receiving palliative and end of life care. This chapter will discuss the sources of such fears, expose any conflicts and offer arguments that explain why this remains the case. The discussion will also look at how death has remained a taboo topic throughout many Western societies. The taboo nature of death can be explained by the unfortunate use of euphemisms around most aspects of death and dying. This chapter will ask you to think through whether euphemisms still have a place in our language and if their use is beneficial, or a hindrance, to our attempts to talk openly about death as articulated in the *End of Life Care Strategy* (DH 2008). It is important that you, and other health care professionals, develop the knowledge and skills necessary to feel confident to care for patients who are receiving palliative and end of life care. In order to do this, you will need to understand the principles that govern the practice of palliative care. The ethos which underpins the delivery of palliative care is central to offering the best care possible to all patients and those deemed important to the patient.

It is true that patients now die in different places, including hospices, hospitals and nursing homes, but most prefer to die in their own home. Why dying in the home is preferred and what could be driving or influencing these decisions will also be discussed. What is important in all aspects of the care and support you offer to patients is that it will improve or enhance their quality of life. Quality of life aims to ensure a dignified and unique death for each patient. There are many reasons why achieving a dignified death is important – one of these is that it helps relatives cope with grief and the bereavement process.

The connection between living and dying

Plants and animals are living things, whereas objects are not: they exist, but are not alive. It is generally thought that only animals (including humans) have consciousness. You are living in the sense that you are thinking, breathing, your heart is pumping blood around your body and your mind is either conscious or unconscious. People are considered to be dying when something threatens their prospect of living, such as terminal illness or acute trauma, but also when they approach old age. When you look closely at this, it is impossible to talk about living without dying and by extension talking about death without considering life as the two are part of the same continuum. Without living, there is no dying and without life there is no death. In addition, life itself is one of those concepts that remains unclearly defined. When does life (living) stop in order for dying to start? Most people would agree that living is the beginning of dying, which in turn signals the end of life. Looking at life and death in this way gives one clue that we cannot separate the two things. In fact one cannot be there without the presence of the other. This cyclical existence only serves to create a complex picture impossible to comprehend. Maybe this could explain why we rarely talk openly about death.

Activity 1.1   *Reflection*

This activity is to allow you time to reflect on how you view life and death and to think about when both life and death begin.

When people are born we like to think that this is when their living starts.

Write down your thoughts about this and say whether you agree with such thinking.

Now write down when you think dying starts. You can include the legal position on death in your country as well as other perspectives you may think of in your writing.

Brief answers to all activities are given at the end of the chapter, unless otherwise indicated. This activity is based on your own observations, so there is no outline answer given.

Your reflections in Activity 1.1 will be unique to you and this will be the same for your patients. However, there are legal positions about when life starts. In the UK it is when a pregnancy is 22 weeks and in the USA it is 20 weeks. The legal positions are not going to be discussed here; the important point for you to think about is whether we can separate living from dying. Nyatanga and Nyatanga (2011) suggest that these two things tend to happen at the same time. The argument they make is that, as you grow from an infant to an adult (living), you are also gradually dying (ageing). You could argue that what we call living is the same as what we call dying because these two aspects/ processes happen at the same time. If you accept this, you can go on to suggest that life is to do with this process (living/dying) and death is in simplistic terms the end of this process.

Most people enjoy their youth and growing up; not many people will consciously think about their dying at the same time. Even people who become ill in their youth rarely consider that they might die. This may in some way explain the absolute horror we feel when a child or young adult dies; our minds are not always prepared for a young person's death. Parents and grandparents often wish roles were reversed and they died instead, and this illogical death of a child makes it hard to 'swallow' for most of us.

This may not be the case in other parts of the world; we see images of death in developing and developed countries, involving both young and old, and due to famine, wars (such as those in South Sudan, Syria or Iraq) and terrorist attacks. We can, wrongly, come to accept their deaths as a consequence of the harsh reality of life through a changing political and environmental landscape. Whether or not it is justifiable, many people find they are more deeply shocked by atrocities involving people they see as being more 'like' them – for example, here in Britain people were shaken by the Bataclan massacre in Paris in 2015, and the attack on people celebrating Bastille Day in Nice the following summer (see *The Guardian* 2016, 15 July). This illustrates a natural tendency to think of disasters as something that happen to 'other people', and the greater power to shock when they happen to people who are relatively close to us in some way. Under normal circumstances, many people living in Western nations do not encounter death in their family until they have reached middle age or beyond. The different experiences we have of living and dying shape our perception of death. The point to remember is that, although death may be the same with regard to how we define it, our perception of it will differ according to individual experiences. Equally, the meaning of death will differ depending on individual expectations in life and in some cases beliefs that we hold about life.

Activity 1.2 — *Reflection*

Reflect on your own perception of death, and then respond to the following points:

- What do you think death is? Write down your thoughts.
- Make a note on aspects of your life that have made you view death in this way, such as religious beliefs, previous experience of death.
- How might your perception of death influence the way you care for patients at the end of their life?

The following part of this activity is optional. If it brings back painful emotional memories or reactions, please feel free not to attempt it.

- Cast your mind back to the very first time you witnessed a human death; write down how old you were at the time. Describe how you think the whole experience affected you and influenced how you feel about death now. Of course, the experience will also depend on who it was that died (whether the person was close to you or not), how the individual died and how old this person was at the time.

As this activity is based on your own observations, there is no outline answer at the end of this chapter.

You might have found Activity 1.2 quite difficult to complete as there is a lack of tangible evidence about what death is really like. Nobody has come back from the dead to tell us about their own experience of death. In addition our perceptions are formed from a range of experiences during our day-to-day life and vary from person to person. It is likely that you have arrived at your perception of death using the experiences of your own life so far. Your perceptions are formed by the things you encounter as you grow up, therefore we can conclude that people are not born with a perception of death. If you agree that people are not born with a perception of death, it follows that these perceptions are learned and are formed by each person as they go through life. You learn things which guide your thinking and behaviour and at the same time you can unlearn things or learn new things that can change your original way of thinking and behaving.

What this suggests is that you and your patients are most likely to have different perceptions of death, and therefore of what death is. Therefore if you are going to help patients with their own dying, you need to understand what death means for them. To do this you need to understand how the patient's history (previous experiences of death) might have shaped the way he or she now views death.

Death as taboo

To delight in talking about death, particularly the prospect of one's own death, is considered morbid in Western society. As a consequence, the topic has become a taboo subject culminating in people fearing death (DH 2008; Nyatanga and Nyatanga 2011). When we consider the possible source of such fear we find explanations in how our young are exposed to death. Even though young children are more likely to be involved in family funerals than they may have been a decade ago, for example, it is much less usual for them to actually see the body. This means that the first time that you encounter death directly might be when you come into nursing. It is perfectly natural to be wary or cautious about something (death) you are not familiar with. Talking openly about it helps make it easier to come to terms with. It becomes a familiar topic to most people, including children, as they grow up. Recognising why people fear death and how this relates to you and your patients will help you to begin to have open conversations with patients and their families, supporting them to face the reality of their situation. The reality here is important and you may have to keep reminding yourself and your patients that, even if we deny death or refuse to talk about it, it will still happen. It is not an option, but a reality for us all.

Fear of death

Most people remain fearful of death and with that we have to argue also that people worry about life. For example, if life was perfect and enjoyable, then most people would like to hold on to it and continue living. Human beings will resist death at any cost; they might pay large sums of money or invest time and resources to preserve life. This would not be the case if life was full of problems, complications and without purpose. There is an inevitable link between life and death in that life with its perpetual problems and complications may make us prefer death as a way of finding an exit point (death-oriented) from life. The opposite is also true: people who love life immensely (life-oriented) will most certainly be fearful of death, because it takes away the very essence of living which they hold dear. Whichever way we look at this we are in fact fearful of death and worried about life. The main difference is that with life you have a choice of what to do, but you rarely have a choice about death and how it comes. This apparent helplessness may explain why most people continue to fear death. In most situations where helplessness is experienced many things happen: the two main ones are loss of control and loss of independence. Dying patients often explain how their disease has made them helpless and unable to fulfil their 'duties' as father, mother, brother, sister or their goals in life including professional potential, social aspirations or global ambitions. It is the loss of these goals and duties that emphasises loss of control and independence for that person. This in turn can promote resentment of the future and fear of death.

Activity 1.3   *Reflection*

Take the time to reflect on what it is about death that makes you fear it. If you do not fear death, reflect on why this is and why some people may fear death. You may wish to discuss this with colleagues or friends.

As this activity is based on your own observations, there is no outline answer at the end of this chapter.

In Activity 1.3 you may have begun your reflection by asking yourself further questions about your fear of death. For example:

- Why is it that people fear death despite the fact that it is a certainty for each and every one of us?
- Even without knowing what lies beyond death (the unknown), why are people still fearful of death?
- Is it at all possible that the unknown itself could be something quite pleasant?

Well done for attempting this activity. These are not easy questions to answer and even philosophers and psychologists have failed to reach unanimous agreement. The philosopher Plato (427–347 BC) presented key points from Socrates' argument about fearing death thus:

> *To fear death, gentlemen, is no other than to think oneself wise when one is not, to think one knows what one does not know. No one knows whether death may not be the greatest of all blessings for man, yet men fear it as if they knew that it is the greatest of evils. And surely it is the most blameworthy ignorance to believe that one knows what one does not know.*

Although Socrates was making a philosophical and logical argument, even now our minds do not seem to be persuaded to stop fearing death, even if we do not fully understand it. There may be many ways of explaining why this remains the case. Some people fear death because it interrupts their life. Death can interrupt a young life, middle-aged life or old life, male or female, rich or poor. Death does not distinguish between black and white, able-bodied or disabled, religious or agnostic and even 'good' and 'bad' people; this makes it indiscriminate and unpredictable (Nyatanga and Nyatanga 2011). If death is not upon us, it is happening elsewhere with someone we know. The media and newspapers are constantly reminding us of death and by extension emphasising how temporary our own life is. This constant reminder makes people more anxious about their life ending and therefore makes them worry more about their death (death anxiety) and that of those most near and dear to us.

The indiscriminate nature of death makes it hard for the human mind to understand how death 'operates'. In life we tend to understand most things, but death is elusive and less predictable. When you look at death in this way, you can begin to see how the irrefutable fact of death creates fear for many people. Medical advances and research have tried to change the course of death, or even avoid it altogether, without success.

Ideas from biology (Brown 2008) give clear guidance that, as one generation grows old, it gives room (through death) for the next one and thereby benefits the species. Biological ideas can only be used to a certain point. The reality of our life is that we spend it growing up well and creating unique identities, working hard, educating ourselves, forming relationships, having desires and gathering possessions – only to be denied all these things by ageing and death.

Our patients are no different from us and they too can experience these realities. Encouraging them to focus on positive experiences could play an important role when we care for dying patients.

Case study

AJ is a 60-year-old life-loving man with strong family values. He was diagnosed with terminal illness two weeks ago when the doctors confirmed cancer of the tongue and gave him up to two years to live. Four weeks ago, AJ had completed his retirement paperwork from his £75,000pa executive job. He was looking forward to spending more quality time with wife Margo of 36 years, and has been saving hard for this, since his three children finished their university education. AJ realizes that the sudden diagnosis and poor prognosis has dramatically changed the future he had anticipated with Margo and his three children, Katie, Binda and Jorpan. The children had just bought them a retirement holiday present for a two-week Mediterranean cruise. The consultant outlined two options for AJ's management.

Option one would include having surgery to remove the affected part of the tongue which would prolong his life by another nine months. Option two would involve no surgery but starting intensive chemotherapy with the hope to shrink the cancer which would add another six months to his life but with 'nasty' side-effects. The consultant also hinted that the cancer may have spread to the lymph nodes, but could not confirm until further tests were performed. AJ has to decide on which option to take within two weeks while he is still asymptomatic in order for the consultant to intervene before the cancer spreads further.

The following activity asks you to consider the situation of AJ from the case study, and attempt to make sense of what you could do to support him and his family to help them to adjust to their new reality. At the moment, the focus is psychological adjustment first and then how to make positive use of the remaining time of AJ's life.

Activity 1.4   *Critical thinking*

- Consider AJ's diagnosis, prognosis and the needs/symptoms he is presenting with, and make a note of what you think AJ's main priority in life is at the moment. You will need to say why you think this is his main priority, and this could be a way of explaining your own judgement of his situation using your nursing or caring skills.
- How would you help and support AJ with his psychological adjustment and his family to cope with his illness? Here you need to think of strategies (psychological) and activities (practical) that you think will help AJ first.

The first part of Activity 1.4 may produce individual judgements of AJ's priorities and you would need to check (confirm) this with AJ himself when you next assess him. Your judgement of his priority may have been influenced by a number of things, including previous experience of caring for someone like AJ or something you once read about as part of your education.

In Activity 1.4 you may have encouraged AJ to weigh up the best option to give him the extra time. It is important to also consider how each option would affect his quality of life. This is important in palliative care as patients may be persuaded by others to take an option that extends their life but leaves them with a very poor quality of life. Of course you would also have thought about AJ opting for the third way, which is not to have anything done and let nature take its course. This would be respecting his choice and you would need to satisfy yourself that AJ was fully aware of the implication of each decision he makes on his quality of life and on family members. It is important to acknowledge the two lives AJ now faces; that is, the life that would have been had he not had this diagnosis, with all the plans post retirement still possible, and the life he now has (the reality) with this cancer that threatens all his plans and goals with Margo and family. AJ will need to readjust to a new reality of existence. The work of Twycross (2003) suggests that it is appropriate to help patients readjust and find new hopes and goals that are in line with their new reality. Twycross calls this achieving reality-based hope and as health care professionals, we can play an important role in making this happen for our patients. However, you should not be surprised if AJ turns to you and asks you to 'help him end it all'. This request is often linked to assisted dying or euthanasia, which are both illegal practices in this country. While being clear and honest with him that you could not help him, you should accompany this with empathy – that is imagining how hard it must be for him to know that his post-retirement plans will not be fulfilled.

It is important that you speak honestly about his situation and the language we use should be clear, without using euphemisms that replace words like dying with 'passing' or 'he is peaceful' when you mean death. These are euphemisms which are discussed in more detail below. After such conversations which are often intense and emotionally charged, make sure you also have support and space to debrief. This is an important aspect of self-care in palliative care which is often ignored when we are busy, and yet it can positively enhance your health and wellbeing.

The role of euphemisms

People try to 'distance' themselves from death by using terms such as 'passed away' or 'passed over' instead of 'died'. Imagine a relative being told that we 'lost' your mum this morning. This message has the potential to confuse and at times relatives misconstrue what is meant. What you have to ask yourself is whether such words (euphemisms) help or hinder our attempts to talk openly and therefore familiarise ourselves with death.

It is common to hear people using euphemisms when referring to death. It is clear that the use of euphemisms does not change the reality of death but somehow offers false and rit-ualistic reassurances which often mask the impulse to panic or temptation to escape from it all. The language of euphemisms tends to convey kindness through words society deems acceptable to describe the dead person. This may also suggest a deep-seated denial or fear of facing up to death. Just like the fear of the possibility of having no further existential (living) possibilities, euphemisms express a pervasive fear of the unknown. You may have heard terms such as 'he has been called to rest', 'she has gone to sleep' or 'he is singing with the angels'. You may have seen RIP written on grave stones or sympathy cards. These euphemisms suggest the dead person is resting in peace and this is seen as being sensitive and more acceptable than saying the person is dead. The fear of death of self and that of loved ones brings about a pseudo-humbleness (softening the harshness of death) and caring expressed through euphemisms. Nyatanga (2008a) claims that the media and in particular newspaper obituaries seem a rich place for these death-related euphemisms. Obituaries are more than cultural rituals. They have a strong social and cultural function for most people (for a more detailed discussion of euphemisms, read Nyatanga 2008a, Chapter 10).

Activity 1.5   *Communication*

This activity asks you to reflect on whether you think euphemisms play a useful role in assisting nurses and health care professionals to face death.

- What terms do you use to avoid saying 'dying', 'dead' or 'death'?
- How do you think the use of euphemisms helps or hinders the way nurses (and other health care professionals) discuss death with their patients or family members?

As this activity is based on your own observations, there is no outline answer at the end of this chapter.

Using euphemisms for death originated with the belief that to speak the word 'death' was to invite death. A common theory holds that death is a taboo subject in most cultures for precisely this reason. We now know that this is an irrational belief, but we continue to hold on to it. In Activity 1.5 you may have stated that euphemisms help soften the impact of death and therefore are a useful tool which shows our sensitive side of caring. Walsh and Nelson (2003) suggest that to be sensitive is the art of saying the same thing in a different way so that we can lessen the hurt or distress death often causes. It is not what you say, but how you say it that makes a difference to the other person. You may also have written about the negative aspects of using euphemisms, especially when misunderstandings may result, and therefore people may not realise death has now occured. An example might result from nurses or doctors saying to relatives, 'We lost your husband this morning', when what they really mean is, 'We are sorry to tell you, your husband died this morning'. It may be said that one is not dying, but *fading away quickly* because *the end is near. Deceased* is a euphemism for dead and sometimes the *deceased* is said to have *gone to a better place.* This is primarily used among the religious with a concept of an afterlife, or heaven.

The tendency for nurses to use euphemisms as a defence mechanism against death anxiety most likely begins with their cultural and religious socialisation. For most people, dependence on parents and society as role models has a lot to do with the eventual inauthenticity and self-deception inherent in euphemisms. First, euphemisms serve to soften the impact of death on family, friends, community and society and also reduce the associated fear of death. Second, euphemisms encourage the portrayal of positive perceptions within a death, focusing on the 'good' aspects of the person who has died. Many people still find death hard to accept and even harder to talk about openly and honestly. Health care professionals often use terms like 'life-threatening disease' or 'life-limiting illness' suggesting our death-denying attitude or simply trying to conform to expectation. It is much harder to say you have a 'death-causing illness'.

Preferred place of care: dying at home

Dying in hospital settings or any institution can present its own challenges as they are not seen as the preferred places for dying by most people. There is evidence (Hunt et al. 2014; Dixon et al. 2016) to suggest that most people would prefer to die in their own home. The question is whether this makes death itself any easier, less feared and more private. Table 1.1 later in the chapter shows a spread of where people prefer to die, and where they actually die.

Before the Industrial Revolution, people died in their own homes surrounded by family and close friends. Aries (1974) made claims that death was very much a private family affair. The suggestion here may be that people saw themselves primarily as part of a family unit and less as individuals, and by extension very much part of a community. Viewing life and death through such a community prism meant that the collective celebration at birth and solidarity in death were important. In this pre-industrial context death was encountered early and we could be right in thinking that many people became familiar with its presence.

Aries claims that the nineteenth century saw a shift of attitudes in favour of *death of the other*. Life and its meaning were now seen through the relationships (personal or intimate) people formed with others. As a result, death was seen as the loss of such relationships. In order for the relationships to develop and flourish, privacy was crucial, if not a prerequisite. Therefore, it followed that any death that took place would no longer be a public event, which means death was no longer being mourned as a loss to the community but a physical separation from a loved one (Nyatanga 2008a).

What followed in the twentieth century was an attitude of *death denied* (Aries 1974). Two things became clear: there were different meanings of death and a sense of cultural belonging. Some cultures wanted to continue with private death, whilst others preferred to share their loss with those important to them. It can be argued that relatives who did not have close relations would end up taking their relative to hospital (or institution) for support and company whilst receiving help with symptom management.

Below is an activity that will allow you to reflect upon your own preferences of where to be cared for and eventually to die. What is important to think about is how much of that decision is entirely yours, and how much is influenced by others, circumstances, and cultural and religious values. We know from the National End of Life Care Intelligence Network (2012) that people do not always die in their preferred place of death. There are many factors to consider when deciding on your preference of place of care, some of which are discussed below. The important point to allude to here is that dying is a process socially engineered by other people, even though there is only one person dying at the time.

Activity 1.6   *Reflection*

Take some time to reflect on the following:

- Where would you like to be cared for (e.g., home, hospital, hospice) and where would you like to be (if different from your first answer) when you die?
- Explain why you have chosen this preference.
- Would your decision be influenced by your family, especially if they did not want you to die in your preferred place of death?
- What might be the impact of where you die on you and your family?

As this activity is based on your own observations, there is no outline answer at the end of this chapter.

The decision of where to be cared for and where to die is left to the patient to make, although in reality, the patient may not have the full range of choices or permission to choose the option. There are many factors to consider when making this decision. For example, whether there is space (that is, beds) in the hospice you prefer, or whether family members also prefer you to die in the family home. Some people may experience difficult and complex symptoms that require hospital/hospice admission for effective management. The home may not have all the medication and equipment needed to control and manage symptoms being experienced. Where there is a mismatch, it affects the dignity of patients.

The idea of dignity is so important to the patient and yet it is least understood by health care professionals. Dignity is about who that person is and ensuring that the care maintains it and at the same time preserves the person's identity. Patients often find themselves struggling to maintain their dignity in the face of aggressive disease that continually erodes their bodies. For example, patients with fungating and odorous tumours struggle to maintain their dignity. Patients can experience social isolation as they face the end of their life, and nurses and other professionals should be there to support them and restore some of their social networks (Astley-Pepper 2005).

There is a large discrepancy between the number of patients who wish to die at home and the actual number that do so (Hunt et al. 2014). It could be argued that families play a part in influencing what happens; indeed, you may have recognised this in your reflection in Activity 1.6. The patient is part of a family unit, so it becomes quite important that their preferences are also shared by the family. The impact of a relative dying at home can have serious consequences, e.g., a family might sell their home because dad died there and they felt uncomfortable living in the house afterwards. Another family might not be able to use the room where their mum died and board it off from the rest of the house. When discussing preferred place of death,

Preferred place of death	Institution as place of care	Actual place of death
3%	HOSPITAL	53%
63%	OWN HOME	21%
29%	HOSPICE	5%
1.50%	CARE HOMES	18%
2.50%	ELSEWHERE	2%
1%	HOME OF RELATIVE OR FRIEND	Unknown

Table 1.1: Summary of places of care and death between 2008/2010
Source: Hunt et al. 2014

consequences like these need to be considered. It is impossible to know in advance what might happen; however, the important point is that we should be aware of these possibilities and find a way of raising them with the family at opportune moments.

Table 1.1 shows the results of a study undertaken to look at where people preferred to die and where they actually died. The study results were reported in 2012 and showed just over 20 per cent of people died in their own home which was their preferred place of death. Although only 3 per cent preferred to die in hospitals, 53 per cent ended up dying there.

The discrepancy in where patients at end of life die and where they want to die tells us that there is more work to be done to ensure that patients receive good palliative care wherever they are being cared for. Some of this work is based in understanding the principles and practice of palliative care. The practice of palliative care is founded in a global philosophy aimed at ensuring that every patient approaching the end of life enjoys an enhanced quality of life.

An overview of the principles and practice of palliative and end of life care

The word 'palliative' can be understood from the English meaning of 'palliate'. The *Compact Oxford English Dictionary* describes 'to palliate' as: *making the symptoms of a disease less severe without curing it* (p731). The main aim is to promote comfort by making symptoms less severe. In practice, the idea of palliative care comes from the Greek word *pallium*, which means to cloak. The symptoms presented by patients with life-threatening illness are *cloaked* (Twycross 2003) with interventions aimed at alleviating the discomfort.

Before the principles of palliative care are discussed we should take time to consider when should, and when does, palliative care begin. Activity 1.7 will give you the opportunity to explore this.

Activity 1.7 | *Critical thinking*

When do you think palliative care should be introduced to patients diagnosed with life-threatening/limiting disease? In your answer state your reasons for the timing.

To help you answer this activity, refer to the book by R.G. Twycross (2003) *Introducing Palliative Care*, 4th edn. Oxford: Oxford University Press and read pages 1–7.

As this activity is based on your own observations, there is no outline answer at the end of this chapter.

As you will have seen, modern thinking suggests that palliative care should start at diagnosis of a life-threatening illness, but other views suggest it should start at a different stage. The original definition offered by the World Health Organization, published in 1990, reflects some of the key points you might have included in Activity 1.7. It states:

> *Palliative care is the active total care of patients with life-limiting disease and their families, by a multi-professional team, when the disease is no longer responsive to curative or life-prolonging treatments.*
> (WHO 1990)

This definition has since been revised in line with new developments and thinking in palliative care to the latest one in 2012, thus:

> *Palliative care is an approach that improves the quality of life of patients and their families facing the problems associated with life-threatening illness, through the prevention and relief of suffering by means of early identification and impeccable assessment and the treatment of pain and other problems, physical, psychological and spiritual.*
> (WHO 2012a)

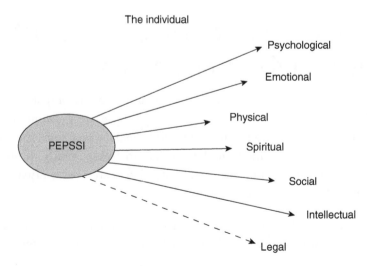

Figure 1.1: The PEPSSI approach to palliative care.

These definitions emphasise the fact that palliative care extends across all dimensions of the patient, not just the physical. Patients may have psychological, social, spiritual, emotional and even intellectual needs, and palliative care aims to address all of them. This approach of caring for all these different aspects of the patient is referred to as total care and is described as the PEPSSI approach (Nyatanga 2008a), as shown in Figure 1.1.

Principles of palliative care

The World Health Organization (WHO) developed eight main guiding principles, listed below. It is important to look at these as *guiding* principles, because their implementation depends on the health care system of each country, the attitudes towards death commonly held and the availability of medicines such as opioids and the many other resources necessary to care for and support patients receiving palliative care.

1. Affirms life and regards dying as a normal process
2. Intends neither to hasten nor postpone death
3. Provides relief from pain and other distressing symptoms
4. Integrates the psychological and spiritual aspects of patient care
5. Offers a support system to help patients live as actively as possible until death
6. Offers a support system to help the family cope during the patient's illness and in their own bereavement
7. Uses a team approach to address the needs of patients and their families, including bereavement counselling, if indicated
8. Will enhance quality of life and may also positively influence the course of illness.

These principles are prone to flaws, but on the whole they serve to equip health care professionals working with dying patients with the knowledge and skills to guide the care of many distressing symptoms. The flaws come when there are different interpretations across the globe. However, two fundamental flaws can be exposed by the contradiction inherent in the first two principles. For example, principle 2 ignores the fact that doctors and nurses interfere with nature before and after birth to protect and prolong life through child immunisation programmes and ongoing treatment for any disease. Yet principle 3 encourages us to provide pain relief without necessarily admitting that some methods of pain relief may also have a negative impact, such as the pain caused by the injection of a pain killer. Although the intention is to control pain, the process may induce pain to eliminate the other pain. Principle 1 encourages people not to regard death as abnormal simply because we do not understand it and, in some cases, fear it.

What is important here is to recognise these difficult and complex issues and you should bear in mind that the care you provide should not discriminate against diagnosis, age, ethnicity or sexual orientation.

The importance of including a team approach is a reflection of the multiple and complex needs of dying patients, which would be impossible for only nurses or doctors to meet. The composition of a typical palliative care team is discussed below. The idea of a team is that 'Together

Everyone Achieves More' (TEAM). This team approach means that the workload and emotional demands of caring for dying patients is shared, thereby protecting each other from excessive stress and even burnout.

Activity 1.8   *Team working*

Palliative and end of life care requires a multidisciplinary team approach. Make a list of all the people you think are part of the multidisciplinary team.

Did you include the patient and family/carers in your list in Activity 1.8? In some situations health care professionals can forget that they are there for the patient and his or her needs. The emphasis in palliative and end of life care on holistic person-centred care indicates that, when the team meets to discuss patient needs, the patient is part of the team. In some situations it is not always possible to have the patient present; therefore it is important that the patient's views are represented. This can be done by talking to the patient before the team meeting or inviting family and carers along. In addition processes such as statements of wishes and preferences and advance care planning can be used to ensure a person-centred focus. See the useful websites section at the end of this chapter for further information about these processes.

When individuals are healthy, they are part of a family unit and are still part of that unit when they become ill and are dying. Caring for the family as well as the patient recognises this fact. Knowing that the family is being cared for reassures patients, allowing them to feel relaxed enough to concentrate their energies on dealing with their symptoms. In the end, when all the principles are followed and implemented properly, Nyatanga (2008a), WHO (2012a), De Souza (2012) and Nyatanga (2016) all suggest these will enhance the quality of life for the dying patient. By extension the principles will achieve a unique and dignified death for the patient, and one that is witnessed by the family.

Where palliative care takes place

There are many settings, such as hospices, hospitals, nursing homes and the community, where palliative care is delivered. While this is true, the key point to remember is that, as a philosophy, palliative care can, and should, be delivered anywhere there is a patient at the end of life. As we have previously discussed in this chapter, the preferred place of care for many dying patients is their own home. However, it is also recognised that this is not always possible. Therefore palliative care should be delivered in any environment where a patient is dying.

Some environments such as hospices are better equipped to care for palliative care patients than others. Therefore it is not surprising that evidence (Thomas 2008; De Souza 2012) tells us that although actual place of death indicates higher numbers dying in hospitals, the preferred place is hospice or home. Hospices offer a range of services. For example, patients with complex symptoms can be admitted to an inpatient unit and have their symptoms controlled. The role of palliative and end of life care in a critical care setting is discussed in Chapter 7.

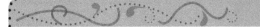

Chapter summary

The idea of living, life, dying and death is intricate and therefore it is not easy to see where each aspect starts and the other ends. It looks like dying starts with the start of living, with the focus more on living in early and healthy life. It is beyond doubt that most people know and probably accept (privately) that one day they will die and yet they find it hard to talk openly about their own death. Most people accept that life and living will one day be interrupted by dying and death, therefore you should encourage open discussion about death and dying with patients who are receiving palliative and end of life care. Open dialogue creates opportunities for the patient and family to say goodbye, mend 'bridges', say sorry for mistakes or misunderstandings, write or rewrite wills. The knowledge that patients are dying can spur them to put their own house in order, make that visit to relatives that they have been putting off and make many other important arrangements. Therefore death can be an unexpected bonus and a platform to make final arrangements in this life. However, dying and death can provoke emotions and anticipatory loss, therefore you should provide effective palliative care that offers support and ensures a dignified death.

Good palliative care should be seen as a philosophy that can be delivered in multiple care settings following the patient on the life journey. Places like hospices can be leading examples for good palliative care, and such exemplars of care should be taken into other settings like hospitals, nursing homes and the community. It is important your care is also extended to the patient's family. They too have needs and concerns. The ultimate goal is to achieve a dignified death free from suffering and an enhanced quality of life.

Finally, caring for people who are dying at the end of life is about the quality of the remaining life and not the quantity. The motto from the Nairobi Hospice captures this concept succinctly:

Put life into their days, and not days into their life.

Activities: brief outline answers

Activity 1.4: Critical thinking

One important fact for AJ to realise and appreciate is how to adjust his wishes and hopes to reflect or be in line with the reality of his own illness. Twycross (2003) talks about the need to ensure that patients do not lose hope about their future aspirations. Instead, they should be encouraged and helped to review their hopes and align them with the demands or difficulties of their illness. In AJ's case, he is going to die within two years and any adjustment and support should take this into account. For example, AJ will need a lot of psychological support to readjust his life to the new realities of his impending non-existence. It is also important when you consider the options available from the consultant and always try and look at the side-effects in view of the overall quality of life for AJ. The requests for assisted dying or euthanasia need a sensitive but honest response. The requests may be signs of psychological 'struggle' within AJ when he may not 'see' the need to carry on with his life and in particular all the pain and suffering that come with the treatment options outlined by the consultant. It is often a patient's wish to control the timing of their death, and sadly the law of the land does not permit this practice. Hopefully, once AJ has come to terms with his prognosis, you also need to help his family understand what it means for AJ so that they too can support him to the end.

Activity 1.8: Team working

You may have included the following in your answer to this activity: specialist nurse, medical doctor, occupational therapist, physiotherapist, pharmacist, dietitian, speech and language therapist (SaLT), complementary therapist, bereavement support worker, educationalist, researcher, chaplain, family support worker, patient, relatives and informal carers.

Further reading

De Vocht, H. and Nyatanga, B. (2007) Health professionals' opposition to euthanasia and assisted suicide: a personal view. *International Journal of Palliative Nursing*, 13 (7): 351–355.

This commentary evaluates the motives of health professionals' opposition to the legislation of assisted dying. It argues that there are justifiable grounds for such opposition in the case of patients who are suffering unbearably and whose request to be helped to die is competent, enduring and voluntary. The authors then engage in plausible speculation about what other, more hidden motives of health professionals might be to reject the legislation of assisted dying. They assert that, while these hidden motives are understandable from a psychological perspective, they also suffocate the self-determination of palliative patients.

Gomes, B., Calazani, N. and Higginson, I. (2011) *Local Preferences and Place of Death in Regions Within England 2010.* London: Cicely Saunders International Centre, Kings College.

This report looked at where people preferred to die and ended up dying within the regions of the UK. It is a useful report as it breaks down the preferences by region and therefore gives readers a more specific picture.

Nyatanga, B. (2015) Making sense of life and death from a death tree. *International Journal of Palliative Nursing*, 21 (10): 473–474.

This commentary is based on ordinary people's thought about death. We asked people during death awareness week to write down their thoughts about death and stick them on a tree we labelled 'death tree'. We then collated all their thoughts and found that there were four different ideas about thoughts which is what is reported in this commentary.

Nyatanga, B. (2016) The essential pillars of palliative care. *British Journal of Community Nursing*, 21 (8): August.

This short article explains the philosophy that underpins the practice of palliative care wherever it takes place.

Nyatanga, L. and Nyatanga, B. (2011) Death and dying. In: Birchenall, P. and Adams, N. (eds) *The Nursing Companion.* Basingstoke: Palgrave Macmillan, pp179–200.

This chapter outlines a lifespan view of death and dying and how society views, copes with and talks about death. It challenges some rituals and practices found in our society and offers explanations of why death is still a difficult topic to discuss openly. The chapter also offers models to help people in the bereavement phase.

Willig, C. (2015) 'My bus is here': a phenomenological exploration of 'living-with-dying'. *Health Psychology,* 34 (4): 417–425.

Useful websites

www.endoflifecare-intelligence.org.uk/resources/publications/

The National End of Life Care Intelligence Network aims to bring all the diverse strands of nationally available data on end of life care together, transform it into intelligence and make this information available in forms which are useful for commissioners, service providers and the public.

http://dyingmatters.org

This is the website for Dying Matters, a broad-based coalition of members whose aim is to change public knowledge and attitudes towards dying, death and bereavement.

www.goldstandardsframework.org.uk/advance-care-planning

This website provides you with information about advance care planning, including links to additional sites.

www.gov.uk/government/uploads/system/uploads/attachment_data/file/536326/choice-response.pdf

This report is in response to an independent review (available at **www.gov.uk/government/publications/ choice-in-end-of-life-care**) of choice in end of life care. It details the six commitments that the UK government has made to the public to end variation in end of life care across the health system by 2020.

Chapter 2
Communication in palliative and end of life care

Jean Fisher

NMC Standards for Pre-registration Nursing Education

This chapter will address the following competencies:

Domain 2: Communication and interpersonal skills

2. All nurses must use a range of communication skills and technologies to support person-centred care and enhance quality and safety. They must ensure people receive all the information they need in a language and manner that allows them to make informed choices and share decision-making. They must recognise when language interpretation or other communication support is needed and know how to obtain it.

Domain 4: Leadership, management and team working

6. All nurses must work independently as well as in teams. They must be able to take the lead in coordinating, delegating and supervising care safely, managing risk and remaining accountable for care given.

NMC Essential Skills Clusters

This chapter will address the following ESCs:

Cluster: Care, compassion and communication

5. People can trust the newly registered graduate nurse to engage with them in a warm, sensitive and compassionate manner.

By the first progression point

3. Interacts with the person in a manner that is interpreted as warm, sensitive, kind and compassionate, making appropriate use of touch.

By entry to the register

8. Listens to, watches for and responds to verbal and non-verbal cues.

9. Engages with people in the planning and provision of care that recognises personalised needs and provides practical and emotional support.

6. People can trust the newly registered graduate nurse to engage therapeutically and actively listen to their needs and concerns, responding using skills that are helpful, providing information that is clear, accurate, meaningful and free from jargon.

By the first progression point
1. Communicate effectively both orally and in writing so that the meaning is always clear.
4. Responds in a way that confirms what a person is communicating.

By entry to the register
8. Communicates effectively and sensitively in different settings using a range of methods and skills.
12. Uses the skills of active listening, questioning, paraphrasing and reflection to support a therapeutic intervention.

Cluster: Organisational aspects of care
14. People can trust the newly registered graduate nurse to be an autonomous and confident member of the multi-disciplinary or multi-agency team and to inspire confidence in others.

By the first progression point
1. Works within the Code (NMC 2015), and adheres to guidance on professional conduct for nursing and midwifery students (NMC 2010).

By the second progression point
2. Values others' roles and responsibilities within the team and interacts appropriately.

Chapter aims

After reading this chapter you will be able to:

- identify, describe and apply the key communication skills required in palliative and end of life care;
- recognise the role 'presence' can have in promoting effective communication in palliative and end of life care;
- understand potential communication barriers in palliative and end of life care and what strategies are available to reduce these.

Introduction

Mel was a 44 year old who, having been very fit and healthy, presented following a sudden major seizure. Investigations established that she had a stage four, very aggressive, brain tumour. When she was given her diagnosis in outpatients clinic she said, 'But you can cure it, right?' The consultant replied, 'I am very sorry to have to tell you that for you cure is not possible.'

Activity 2.1   *Reflection*

Using the quote above and your own experience, think about and make brief notes on communication issues in palliative and end of life care situations that give you cause for concern. These may be issues you have encountered or witnessed, or things that you anticipate will be difficult if and when they arise. Consider why these particular scenarios concern you.

Brief answers to all activities are given at the end of the chapter, unless otherwise indicated. This activity is based on your own observations, so there is no outline answer given.

Although traditionally seen as being focused on cancer (Radbruch 2011), palliative and end of life care is a crucial component of long term conditions management, e.g., motor neurone disease (MND). Palliation may be needed for adults from the point of diagnosis of advanced disease, be that cancer or a non-malignant condition, or subsequent to a severe trauma or stroke. Recent publications including Leadership Alliance for the Care of Dying People (2014) and Department of Health (2016) and guidance such as National Council for Palliative Care (2015) and NICE (2015) have highlighted the need for excellence in communication as part of the provision of end of life care. Effective, person-centred communication in palliative and end of life care is relevant whether we care for pregnant or nursing mothers, a child with severe disabilities or a progressive illness, or elderly people with dementia.

Communication is at the heart of your nursing practice, and is the core of *The Code: Professional standards of practice and behaviour for nurses and midwives* (NMC 2015). The above quote and your reflection in Activity 2.1 highlight the complexity of the situations encountered in palliative and end of life care. Developing your knowledge and skills and exploring communication in palliative and end of life care will increase your confidence in this area and will support you to provide person-centred care. Effective communication enables you to assess pain and other symptoms accurately; to explore issues and concerns; to offer comfort and support to the dying person and his or her family and friends. Communication skills are pivotal to achieving true multidisciplinary practice in any arena of health care, and never more so than when you are caring for the very ill, the dying and the bereaved.

Fundamental components of communication in palliative and end of life care

There are many constituents of communication; however the work of Mehrabian (1967) identified three central ingredients within the 'communication cake': facial expressions and body language, the way the words are spoken and the words that are spoken and that, for white Anglo-Saxons, body language is such a significant aspect that it represents more than half (55 per cent) of the message conveyed. Body language consists of eye contact, body position

Element of body language	Potential message conveyed
Eye contact (EC)	Little EC may be seen as lack of interest. Too much EC can be threatening and in some situations is better avoided, for example, some people with autistic spectrum disorder may find eye contact deeply distressing.
Posture (P)	Closed P (crossed legs/arms etc.) may convey unfriendliness or rejection whereas an open relaxed P suggests warmth and friendliness. Drooped head and shoulders may indicate depression or despair; muscular tension and stiffness can be signs of anxiety.
Facial expression (FE)	FE conveys both emotion and attitudes. For people who cannot use facial expression, e.g., those with Parkinson's disease, opportunities to convey messages are compromised.
Gestures (G)	G can be used to reinforce or emphasise certain points. Remember some people use gesticulation and shoulder shrugging much more. Furthermore, when caring for people from minority ethnic groups it is vital to consider how your non-verbal communication may be interpreted differently and the effect this might have on your relationship with that person.

Table 2.1: Body language and its significance in communication

and openness, e.g., whether your arms are crossed or relaxed by your side (Mehrabian 1967). In some cultures and countries body language may be more or less significant, e.g., the Italians utilise body language and hand gestures more than people in the UK. Crosscultural significance of gestures can also differ: in Tibet the sticking out of the tongue is a greeting and is not considered to be rude. Table 2.1 summarises aspects of body language and their potential significance in communication.

The way the words are spoken, your tone, represents over one-third of communication and can have a profound impact on how what you are saying is received; is your tone harsh, encouraging, loud or soft? Finally, the words spoken account for only a small part of your communication (7 per cent). However, the words you choose can mean more depending on whether the communication is face to face, and on the level of understanding a person has, e.g., when a patient has cognitive decline. Ensuring that your words are not ambiguous is vitally important: in palliative and end of life care, using terms such as 'passed away' instead of 'died' may cause confusion at a time of emotional distress.

Mehrabian (1967) identified these proportions from research specifically in relation to feelings and attitudes, and he did not intend them to be seen as absolute or applying in all situations. The congruence of messaging between the three ingredients is of significant importance. If your words convey one message but your tone and body language convey another, then the message received may be mixed, or confused. For example, 'I am really sorry to hear about your mother's death' could be stated with clear eye contact and a warm tone. This would signal a genuine response.

However, the same words spoken in a dismissive tone and/or whilst looking at your watch demonstrate to the listener that actually you do not really care and/or that you are distracted by something else which you perceive as more important.

In a face-to-face conversation with a patient and/or family, when the words you use are perhaps less significant than you think, there is a high need for congruence in terms of your body language and tone. This is to ensure a clear and consistent meaning is received and understood by the person you are communicating with. However not all communication takes place face to face and you need to consider the implications of this for your practice.

Case study

Maria is a widow with advanced renal failure. She is in the ward where you are working and is expected to die very soon. Her daughter Claudia has been visiting daily and you know they are very close. They moved from Romania ten years ago and have no relatives in the UK. Claudia has said she wants to be with her mum when she dies, but unfortunately Maria deteriorates very suddenly and dies without her daughter present. Your mentor asks you to phone Claudia at work and give her the news of her mother's death.

Activity 2.2   *Communication*

Reflecting on the case study and considering the fundamental aspects of communication, answer the following:

- How would you feel about making this telephone call?
- What factors would you take into consideration?
- What fundamental aspects of communication would you need to pay attention to particularly in respect of how you communicate this news?
- How might the conversation be different if you were talking face to face with Claudia?

In Activity 2.2 you may have reflected on the difficulty of not being able to see Claudia when breaking this news to her. We interpret and deduce much from people we are communicating with by *their* body language and tone too. This may explain why many nurses and other health care professionals find telephone interactions in the context of palliative and end of life care difficult. In that situation you are much more reliant on the words you use and how you say them. In addition you cannot see the person's body language to judge how he or she is reacting to the news. You need to rely on the individual's words and silences to gauge his or her response.

You may also have reflected on the fact that not being present at the time of the death may impact on Claudia's subsequent bereavement (see Chapter 3). Similarly the fact that there are no other family members locally may affect Claudia's ability to cope well in bereavement.

Touch in palliative and end of life care

Touch is an important aspect of non-verbal communication. In Activity 2.2, were Claudia to have been present you might well have used touch to convey empathy. Touch is an important communication tool to use when undertaking complex and difficult conversations. Touch can convey what sometimes we would struggle to put meaningfully into words. However, as a nurse, you must learn to use touch when needed and appropriate for the individual, rather than having a blanket one-size-fits-all approach. There are many cultural and societal aspects that you need to recognise and respect when considering the use of touch. Using touch can support and enable communication, but it is crucial to remember it can also act as a blocking technique (see section on barriers to effective communication). As a nurse you may well be more comfortable with touch than some of the patients you support and care for. When you touch a patient/family member it should be because you believe it will help that person, not because the touch helps you feel more comfortable.

It is important to remember that for some individuals the only touch they receive is when a carer is giving physical care. This could be described as a technical form of touch, but as Clarke (2013) highlights, the way in which you touch a patient when undertaking even the simplest of care procedures such as taking a person's blood pressure will communicate much about your attitudes and beliefs about your work and your patient. Your touch can help or hinder the building of the vital relationship between you and your patient. Often the most intimate aspects of personal physical care can create opportunities for very deep connections and meaningful communication, but only if our touch is thoughtful and based on kindness and compassion.

Communication without words

For people with dementia common methods of communication can become more difficult over time. Much has been written about the importance of joining the person with dementia in their world, rather than causing distress through reorientation to the here and now (Blackhall et al. 2011). More recently Simard (2013) has described the value of making connections and enhancing quality of life for those with advanced dementia through Namaste care. This programme of care involves regular short periods of sensory stimulation, the use of music and sounds, therapeutic touch, colour, food treats and scents. All of these elements are ways of connecting and communicating with a person for whom speech may no longer have so much, if any, meaning. Although the programme itself can appear complex, elements of it can easily be incorporated into everyday nursing practice. Simply stroking the hand is a way of conveying that we care about the person with dementia and may calm and soothe them. Playing music that has meaning for the individual can be equally helpful and can involve family members in creating a play list of old favourites. The work of Stacpoole et al. (2014) has highlighted therapeutic benefits of the strategies within Namaste care, including the lessening of some behavioural symptoms and distress, and the use of these simple techniques in communicating with the person with advanced dementia.

Watch the YouTube clip 'Old man in nursing home reacts to hearing music from his era': **www.youtube.com/watch?v=NKDXuCE7LeQ** and, reflecting on this and the paragraph above on Namaste care, consider how you can integrate simple techniques of communicating without words into your practice with individuals with dementia. You may wish to consider those elements that involve family and staff working together to bring comfort and pleasure to the person with dementia

As this activity is based on your own reflection and thoughts, there is no outline answer at the end of this chapter.

Key facilitative skills to support communication in palliative and end of life care

A basic principle that underpins all interactions with a patient who is facing the end of life, or with a family member or a close friend, is for you to find out the person's areas of concern. You will then use this information to focus fully on their needs. There are a number of facilitative skills that support and enable this approach. Table 2.2 discusses these and the context for their use.

You can practise the facilitative skills in Table 2.2 and over time they will become embedded within your nursing practice. However there may be times when you feel out of your depth; when you are unable to answer a question or how to address a concern expressed by a patient or family member. This might be when a patient or relative asks you a difficult question outright.

Key facilitative skills (Goldberg et al. 1993; Zimmerman et al. 2003; Maguire et al. 1996)	Examples and contexts for use in palliative nursing practice
Open questions (OQ), open directive questions (ODQ)	*OQ*: 'How are you feeling?' As this question is very wide it enables the person to decide what to focus on and how much to tell you. *ODQ*: 'Tell me about your pain?' This provides a more specific focus for the response but is still not overly prescriptive.
Acknowledging (A) Reflecting (R) Paraphrasing (P)	*A* is a skill that allows us to demonstrate that we recognise the situation the person has shared with us. *R* enables us to use patients' words back to them to show we have heard them, e.g., 'You felt really upset ...'

	P allows us to use their words in a way which demonstrates our listening and comprehension: 'You found that time really painful.'
	Often use of these skills will encourage patients to tell us more about their feelings because we have demonstrated our interest.
Checking/clarifying (C/Cl)	*C/Cl* can help you to identify if you are getting the gist of what you are being told accurately.
Summarising (S)	*S* can help us to demonstrate we have been listening attentively: 'So you said that things have been going quite well but you have been concerned about your mother and also the increase in your neck pain, especially in the mornings.'
	We can also ask patients/family members to *S*, as a way to check out what they know or have taken in. 'Can you tell me what you have been told so far about your illness?' NB: This is a better way of putting this question than: 'What can you remember about what they told you about your illness?' – you get what they remember but without them feeling the pressure of remembering it.

Table 2.2: Key facilitative skills and their use in palliative and end of life care

Scenario

Imagine you are nursing Mrs Jill Cox, who has advanced multisystems atrophy and is unable to communicate verbally. Her brother Philip comes to see her. He meets you in the corridor and asks you, 'Is Jill dying?'

Activity 2.4   *Critical thinking*

Using the information in Table 2.2, consider what key facilitative skills you would use in this situation. Use the following points to guide your discussion:

- Do you know how much information Jill is happy for Philip to have about her condition?
- What open and open directive questions might you ask Philip?
- What would you say to acknowledge how Philip is feeling at this time?
- How would you reflect back to Philip what he is feeling?

At times like the situation in Activity 2.4 you may not know the answer to the questions posed. You may refer on to another colleague or seek guidance and then speak with the person again. If you do not know the answer it is acceptable to say: 'I'm sorry, Philip, but I don't know the answer to your question.' If you express empathy and concern for him, and offer alternative help to explore his questions, you will have recognised the concern expressed and addressed that. It may have taken Philip a huge amount of courage to express his concern. The crucial thing is not to ignore, or worse still, to dismiss it.

The role of silence in communication in palliative and end of life care

Additional to the key skills already mentioned, the use of silence is known to enable and facilitate communication (Eide et al. 2004). Pauses, particularly in the context of breaking bad news or other difficult conversations, help your patients by giving them time to think through what has already been said. Remember, when people are ill, frail or in distress, it may take longer for them to process information anyway. Pauses will aid people to consider if they wish to ask a question, or not; if they can trust you, or not; and to consider how they are feeling about what has already been said. Although it may seem silent to you, there will usually be much 'internal dialogue' going on in the mind of the patient. Of course silence can sometimes help you too as it gives you a moment to think, or 'catch your breath'. Maintaining a pause in the conversation is often very difficult; your natural instinct might be to speak and 'fill the void'. Enabling a pause often leads the person to talk more. However, if the pause becomes uncomfortable for them, try to find a way to encourage them to speak. Try to avoid filling the silence simply to avoid your own discomfort, but in order to enable them to express themselves. Perhaps you could ask them gently if they can tell you what they are thinking. Be aware though that sometimes thoughts can be too difficult to put into words and if the person does not want to talk, then respect that. It may be that you revisit this with them at a later date.

The use of cues and educated guesses in palliative and end of life care

A cue is when a person gives a hint, verbal or non-verbal, that suggests an underlying emotion. A cue provides you with an opportunity to explore and clarify what the person has alluded to in the cue (Del Piccolo et al. 2006). If you are actively listening and responding appropriately to the presented cues then the person is far more likely to open up and tell you more about the situation, fears and concerns. A sigh, a frown or a half-expressed thought may all be cues; for example, a tailed-off sentence: 'Lately I've been wondering ...' When patients use cues, this is an opportunity for you to use the key facilitative skills to explore with them their concerns and to provide them with information or advice or simply the opportunity to talk.

Educated guesses are used to try to interpret what has happened or what the person has already told you, and to demonstrate sensitive listening. Educated guesses should always be offered tentatively. You do not want to assume that you know what the person is thinking or feeling, or that you are putting words into their mouth. Educated guesses are often prefaced by a phrase such as 'It sounds as if ...' or 'It seems like that might ...'. Consider these two statements made by a nurse when a patient disclosed that, as a teenager, he had looked after his dying mother:

- 'That must have been very difficult for you.'
- 'It sounds like that might have been really hard for you.'

The first statement assumes that it could not have been anything other than very difficult to do this and it is likely therefore that the patient will agree with this. In the second statement you can sense the nurse is not assuming anything. In reality the patient may have been pleased to care for his mother, and may not have felt that it had been hard. The second statement enables him to say, 'Yes, it was really tough ...' or 'I loved her, so although it wasn't easy ...'. This may then lead to further information being disclosed which may help us to offer appropriate care in the future.

Case study

Mike is 36. He lives with his partner Chloe and their two children aged 11 and 9. Chloe works part time in a shop. Mike has lung cancer and advancing COPD, secondary to his use of cannabis. During your work in primary care you are asked to accompany your mentor to undertake an assessment visit to see Mike at home. He is quiet and seems very anxious. During the visit he suddenly says, 'How long will it be?'

Activity 2.5   *Critical thinking*

Consider Mike's case study above. How might you use some of the specific skills already discussed in this chapter to help find out what concerns and issues Mike may be worrying about?

Activity 2.5 will have highlighted the importance of using skilled communication to support the assessment of a patient and his needs. It would be easy to ignore Mike's concerns and undertake an assessment that overlooks these. You cannot assume what is uppermost in Mike's mind, e.g., his children, financial concerns or spiritual concerns. The important thing is that you assess rather than assume.

Presence in palliative and end of life care

Your role in this part of a patient's life may be for just a few hours or for many months. Palliative and end of life care can occur in any setting, e.g., critical care unit, hospice or care home. The foundations of palliative care were discussed in Chapter 1. Many skills, encompassing both 'the science' of nursing, e.g., pain management, and 'the art' of nursing, e.g., communication, are needed to provide compassionate care which maintains dignity and upholds autonomy in the face of increasing dependence and significant uncertainty. The care you provide will not only impact on the person who is dying but can have a major influence on the coping and bereavement of the family members, and therefore their future health and wellbeing.

The Francis Report (2013) into failings at the Mid Staffordshire NHS Foundation Trust identified a lack of compassion, at all levels within the trust, as a contributing factor to the neglect patients experienced. Nouwen (1982: 121) says compassion *asks us to go where it hurts, to enter into the places of pain, to share in brokenness, fear, confusion and anguish ... compassion means full immersion in the condition of being human.* You might find this quote quite challenging; immersing yourself in someone else's pain and fear can be quite daunting. Developing your own *emotional resilience* will aid delivery of compassionate care and your own emotional wellbeing. In 2012 the Chief Nursing Officer identified compassion as one of the 'six Cs' (Commissioning Board Chief Nursing Officer and DH Chief Nursing Adviser 2012). Here compassion is encompassed with care: *compassion is how care is given through relationships based on empathy, respect and dignity – it can also be described as intelligent kindness, and is central to how people perceive their care.* This is, perhaps, a more accessible definition and places compassion in terms of communication and the therapeutic relationship you develop with your patients.

In palliative and end of life care communication and demonstrating compassion are not solely focused on verbal communication. Nouwen (1982) discusses the 'ministry of presence' and how being with someone can, of itself, be powerful, useful and therapeutic. Presence is a way of 'being' with a patient, encompassing behaviours that express caring and compassion. These include being sensitive and aware of the person and his or her needs, being attentive and focusing on the patient and his or her needs and connecting with them as a person (Covington 2003). 'Being with' patients reaffirms to them that you value them and you are there for them; your presence may reassure them during a difficult procedure, or support them to make a difficult decision (Covington 2003). Presence and 'being with' a patient focuses on the very heart of your relationship with your patient. It encompasses compassion, communication, spirituality and person-centred care.

Activity 2.6 — *Reflection*

Reflecting back on your clinical experience to date, think of a situation when you have witnessed a nurse, or other health care professional, using presence as a therapeutic and nursing intervention. Consider the following points:

- Could you identify when presence was used? What indicated this to you?
- How did the nurse demonstrate 'presence'?
- How did this support the nurse to engage with the patient on an interpersonal and spiritual level?
- What was the effect of this on the patient?
- What was the effect of this on the nurse?

The article by Wilson (2008) listed in the further reading section will provide you with further information to use in this activity.

As this activity is based on your own observations, there is no outline answer at the end of this chapter.

Activity 2.6 will have enabled you to consider presence and how it is used in palliative and end of life care as an effective communication method. You should not always assume, however, that at times of distress or when they are close to death, patients value having family members, other loved ones or a member of staff close by. Nouwen (1982) also suggests that for some, at particular times, absence can be as useful or necessary as presence. Knowing which approach to use relies on you having developed a positive therapeutic relationship with your patient, and his or her family or carer.

Barriers to effective communication in palliative care

Barriers to communication can exist either on the part of the patient/family member or the health care professional. Potential barriers to communication can take many forms, e.g., sensory impairment. You can use simple strategies, ensuring patients have their glasses on, and hearing aid in place and switched on. These will make a significant difference to their hearing and thus comprehension of any conversations that take place. Those who are not obviously deaf may have some hearing deficit. Most people use lip reading to a degree, even though we may not be aware of it. So consideration of your position and the person being able to see your face when you speak is also important. Patients with a neurological condition, e.g., Parkinson's disease, may lose their ability to use facial expressions to display emotion. Patients may be frightened to ask questions about their future – they may not want to hear the answer.

You may put up your own barriers to communication by avoiding eye contact with patients, engaging them in 'small talk' or avoiding answering their questions (Maguire et al. 1996). To ensure effective and positive communication it is important that you recognise and understand the potential barriers that may be present, both in your patients and yourself. Gaining an insight into why your patients, and you, might create barriers will also promote patient-centred communication. In addition, recognising why you might 'block' communication will support the development of your emotional intelligence.

Two useful frameworks have been developed to support health care professionals in recognising why patients and health care professionals may put up barriers to communication. These can be remembered by the acronyms FEARS (fears, environment, attitudes, responses, skills) and FIBS (fears, inadequate skills, beliefs, support) (Tables 2.3 and 2.4). FEARS is used for potential patient barriers and FIBS is used for possible barriers present in you and other health care professionals.

FEARS element	Manifestation
Fears	Being judged as ungrateful; being stigmatised; crying/breaking down; burdening/causing distress to the health professional.
Environment	Lack of privacy; person present or absent who needs to be/not be there with me.
Attitudes	This person does not have time to listen to me, or it is not this person's job to talk about this; my concerns are not important; I should be able to cope with this; my family would not want me to talk about this.
Responses (from health care professionals)	Distanced or disengaged; relevant questions were not asked of me; being touched when I need my own space.
Skills	I cannot find the right words/have not sufficient command of language/do not understand enough to know what to ask; literacy levels; mental capacity issues.

Table 2.3: FEARS: potential patient barriers to communication

FIBS element	Manifestation
Fears	Causing upset or harm; emotional responses; saying 'the wrong thing'; being asked difficult questions; taking too much time.
Inadequate skills	Lack of assessment skills for psychological issues and concerns as well as physical ones; inability to integrate physical and non-physical agendas together into a full holistic review.
Beliefs	Emotional problems are inevitable in serious/life-threatening illnesses; nothing can be done about them so it is pointless to bring up issues we 'cannot solve'; it is 'someone else's role to do this'.
Support	Lack of support for the patient if problems are identified; feeling professionally unsupported; team conflicts.

Table 2.4: FIBS: possible barriers in health care professionals

Activity 2.7   *Reflection*

Reflecting back on your clinical practice, think of a situation where you found communication with a patient or relative difficult or challenging. Using the FEARS and FIBS frameworks, consider what patient barriers may have impacted on the interaction and recognise what may have inhibited your ability to communicate effectively.

As this activity is based on your own observations, there is no outline answer at the end of this chapter.

Considering your own practice in relation to the above barriers should help you to be more aware of them in the future and to be able to address them in a constructive way.

There is significant evidence that people find it helpful to discuss their fears and concerns. There is not always an expectation or need for 'an answer'. However, the barriers you identified in Activity 2.7 as impacting on your ability to communicate with people in difficult situations may prevent you from 'walking on dangerous ground'. Your concerns may prevent you from offering the person the opportunity to talk. This in turn may lead to their concerns and needs not being expressed or met. You may not always be able to prevent some of the barriers within yourself; however the more self-aware you are the more likely you are to work actively to address these barriers. Similarly, if you can be mindful of the types of issues which can hinder communication from the patient/carer perspective you may be able to use your own skills to mitigate against these. Skilful and empathic assessment to find out the worries and concerns the person is really experiencing and seeing things from that person's angle will of itself be beneficial, even if you cannot 'offer an easy solution'.

Complex communication in palliative and end of life care

Tuffrey-Wijne and McEnhill (2008) have noted the particular difficulties that caring for someone with a learning disability at end of life can pose. The *Route to Success* document (NHS Improving Quality 2015) sets out ways to enhance care at end of life for this group of people. As a nurse you need to be aware of the particular complexities around truth telling and decision making. You will need to seek appropriate support to be able to offer the best possible opportunity for your patient to make his or her own decisions, or to have as much involvement as possible. Read (2006) reminds us that for some family members the idea of autonomy for the person with the learning disability can be very hard. We have a responsibility to support family members who may already have suffered multiple losses in relation to this person.

Case study

Pauline is 59. She has Down's syndrome and Alzheimer's disease, characterised by an increasingly impaired memory and unusual restlessness. She lives in a small care home with three other residents and she seems happy there. Pauline's father died in hospital whilst he was recovering from minor abdominal surgery. Although she was very upset at the time Pauline seems to have coped well since and rarely mentions her dad, although she has repeatedly said she hates hospitals. Her mother Susan visits her regularly and her two older brothers help Susan to take Pauline out at least once a month, which she enjoys. Pauline attends a day centre and has a busy social life with her friends, particularly going to music events.

Pauline was diagnosed with type 2 diabetes two years ago. She also has COPD. She has been admitted to hospital twice in the past six months because of recurrent chest infections. On her last admission she required two courses of intravenous antibiotics to eradicate the infection. This caused her great distress as she could not easily get up and around. She has said several times that she 'never wants to go back in hospital ever again, not even if I dies'.

The care home staff are all very fond of Pauline. She has been in their care for almost a year. She is a warm and friendly woman who loves fun and laughter. The staff have expressed concern to the GP about Pauline saying she does not want to go into hospital again if she needs treatment. They have tried to discuss this issue with Susan but she is adamant that Pauline must be readmitted if necessary. Susan refuses to discuss or even mention the matter with Pauline.

Things come to a head when a new senior carer starts working at the care home. She tries to talk with Susan about Pauline's expressed wishes not to return to hospital. Susan becomes very angry and says that if the staff do not do as she asks she will sue the care home as they have no right to discuss things with Pauline as she, Susan, is Pauline's mother.

Activity 2.8	Decision-making

You are accompanying the community nurse (Valerie) who is offering support to the care home team and helping to monitor Pauline's diabetes and COPD for the primary health care team. Pauline and Valerie have known each other for two years and have built up a good relationship. Pauline always refers to 'Valerie the vampire', and although you know she does not enjoy having blood tests done she has never refused them, as she says it helps her be able to have some sweeties sometimes. The care home phone and ask for help in talking with Susan.

Using the information in this chapter, consider the following:

- What potential barriers to communication is Susan displaying?
- What key facilitative communication skills could you use to explore these with Susan?
- Who might you consider including in any conversations?

Activity 2.8 will have allowed you to relate some of the key principles of communication to a case study, in addition to considering effective communication in this case study, as well as issues around whether Pauline has capacity to make decisions for herself. Issues of consent in palliative and end of life care are discussed further in Chapter 8. Given the complexity of this situation Susan will need a significant amount of support throughout. The relationship that you make as a nurse with her is deeply important to being able to offer that support. Balancing upholding Pauline's rights and Susan's needs may cause tension and difficulties. In these kinds of situation the person often 'has an inkling' of the truth of the situation and is looking to us to confirm the reality rather than the news being a 'bolt out of the blue'. It is important to remember that confidence is much harder to regain once lost, and that all the team may be mistrusted once one team member is considered to be dishonest.

In situations where a child or young person is very ill, communication is at the centre of ensuring person-centred care. Review the case study below and then consider the questions that follow.

Case study

Joe is 15. He has Duchenne muscular dystrophy. He can still stand and take some steps with help but knows he will soon need a wheelchair. Although his parents have told him that he has a progressive condition, they have not told him that this condition will shorten his life very significantly. Pete is a staff nurse working in the ward where Joe has been admitted with a chest infection. Joe responds quite well to intravenous antibiotics, and within a couple of days is chatting to Pete about his favourite football team. During this conversation Joe asks Pete what Pete thinks about having to be in a wheelchair a lot of the time. Whilst Pete is considering his response to this Joe says, 'My Mum says there will be a cure for me soon, but I am not sure. I don't think I want to spend the next fifty or more years in a chair.' Pete is shocked and does not know how to respond to this statement. Joe looks at him and says, 'Oh don't worry Pete I am sure she will be right in the end, do you think Chelsea will win the cup this season?'

Activity 2.9   *Critical thinking*

Using the information and the knowledge you have gained in reading this chapter, consider the following points:

* What key facilitative communication skills could Pete use in this situation?
* What barriers may Pete be presenting to effective communication?
* What might be the consequences of Pete not telling Joe the truth?
* Why do you think Joe may have replied as he did?

The case study in Activity 2.9 has the potential to be particularly challenging; you may have included some of these challenges in your answers to the questions posed. Not only did Pete have to consider key aspects of communication but he also had to recognise the legal issues of open dialogue with a minor without parental presence (see Chapter 8 for further information regarding this).

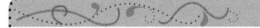

Chapter summary

Within this chapter we have considered the various helps and hindrances to effective communication in the context of palliative and end of life care. The value of a therapeutic relationship has been the thread throughout, together with the acknowledgement of the emotional cost to you as a nurse of investing in such relationships with people facing loss and death. By using the skills discussed and being present and mindful in your interactions you will help not only your patients and those close to them, but also yourself to become richer and more rounded, both as a person and as a practitioner.

Activities: brief outline answers

Activity 2.2: Communication

This is a common scenario that you will meet in practice. Issues you might have wanted to consider in advance include:

- Had anyone explained to Claudia that there might not be any warning of Maria's death and that it might not be possible for her to be present if something happened suddenly?
- Are there any cultural considerations to take into account for Maria or Claudia?
- Did the notes give details of friends that you could contact (with Claudia's permission) to be with her after you had broken the news of Maria's death? What support might she be able to gain through her workplace if any?
- What issues may there be if Maria had expressed a wish to be buried back home in Romania?

Aspects you might have included were that you would find it more difficult to speak to Claudia over the phone than face to face, because you would not find it easy to gauge her responses to you without the benefit of her body language. You would need to pay special attention to your tone as this would convey your compassion and empathy.

Activity 2.4: Critical thinking

- Open question: 'What has prompted you to ask this question?' Open direct question: 'Has something changed in Jill's condition that makes you think this?'
- 'That's a difficult question to ask. You must be quite worried about Jill.'
- 'I can see you find this difficult to talk about. Would you like to go somewhere quiet where we can discuss this?'

Activity 2.5: Critical thinking

In this kind of conversation your tone and body language will be crucial in conveying your willingness to talk openly with Mike.

- Clarifying the time available for the conversation may be a helpful starting point for both of you. It will be difficult for him to 'open up' if he knows his partner will be coming home in the next few minutes, or if he expects that you have only five minutes to spend with him. This is an approach that some practitioners find difficult, but in most care contexts patients are used to an unspoken time-frame of five to ten minutes, so hearing that you have more than this to offer could be very positive and create an openness and equality in the relationship from the outset.
- In addressing Mike's question it will be essential first to clarify what he means by his question. He might mean long until the disease progresses or until he dies – but he might mean until the family return. The use of very gentle reflection and echoing his words '… be long until … ?' will offer him the chance to tell you what he means by that question, or indeed to decide he does not want the answer and therefore he may change the subject.
- Using open questions such as 'How are things for you at present?', or 'What are the most important issues for you right now?' will enable Mike to choose what to focus on, and may lead to further disclosure.

Activity 2.8: Decision-making

Things you might usefully have included in your answer are as follows:

- Susan might present the following barriers to communication. F (fears): Susan may be afraid that because Pauline has a learning disability she will not be offered optimum care. She might be frightened she will cry and that she will burden the staff in the care home. A (attitudes): Susan may think she has the right to make decisions on Pauline's behalf or that she should be able to cope with this. S (skills): Susan may feel that she does not understand enough about Pauline's health to be involved in a discussion like this. In addition Susan may wish to protect Pauline.
- Acknowledging how Susan is feeling about this situation will help validate her feelings. The use of open and open direct questions will allow you to explore in more detail why Susan is reluctant to discuss future care needs with Pauline. Reflecting and paraphrasing back to Susan will encourage her, with your support, to explore her feelings behind her decision.
- Others you will need to involve include the GP, care home staff, and additionally the Community Learning Disability Team, who may help to offer advice and support. If necessary a referral to the Independent Mental Capacity Advocacy service can also be made.

Activity 2.9: Critical thinking

Key aspects and issues in this situation relate to both Joe's pre-existing knowledge and insight into his illness.

- It would be useful to find out what information Joe had previously been given and what he understood from that, as well as what information his parents are happy for him to have, particularly as they were not present at the time he asked the question. Knowing what Joe's parents know and understand and the level of openness there is between them all about the disease and the future is fundamental, not only to effective communication, but also to offering supportive family-focused care.
- Pete could have used both open and open directive questions to find out why Joe had spoken as he did. Doing this would have allowed further exploration of Joe's thoughts and feelings in more detail. Reflecting back and clarifying information would have ensured Pete understood what it was that Joe was asking about the wheelchair use.
- Pete could have presented the following barriers. F (fear): he might have been frightened to discuss this further with Joe; he might have not wanted to risk upsetting him. I (inadequate skills): Pete may not feel he has the necessary skills to discuss this; Joe's age could be a contributing factor.

- If Pete had not told the truth then it seems very likely that Joe would have lost faith in him as a nurse.
- Joe's response may have been because he genuinely thought that his mother's belief in cure could be achieved. However it could be that Pete's expression told him the truth, and he did not need words to confirm it. An alternative reason for him replying thus is that he may have been trying to spare Pete's feelings. He might have felt sorry for having asked this difficult question, as patients sometimes do.

Further reading

Baughan, J. and Smith, A. (2013) *Compassion, Caring and Communication: Skills for Nursing Practice.* Harlow: Pearson.

This text explores the interconnectedness of three core components of excellence in nursing care.

Kabat Zinn, J. (2011) *Mindfulness for Beginners: Reclaiming the Present Moment and Your Life.* Boulder, CO: Sounds True.

This text provides an introduction to mindfulness, a practice derived from Buddhist teachings.

Wilson, M.H. (2008) 'There's just something about Ron': one nurse's healing presence amidst failing hearts. *Journal of Holistic Nursing,* 26 (4): 303–307.

Useful websites

http://dyingmatters.org

This website focuses on raising awareness about dying, death and bereavement. There are useful resources about how to talk to people about death and dying.

See also the below YouTube clips about touch, music and validation therapy in dementia.

'Gladys Wilson and Naomi Feil'

'Alive Inside': How the magic of music proves therapeutic for patients with Alzheimer's and dementia.

Chapter 3
Exploring loss, grief and bereavement

Jane Nicol

NMC Standards for Pre-registration Nursing Education

This chapter will address the following competencies:

Domain 1: Professional values

9. All nurses must appreciate the value of evidence in practice, be able to understand and appraise research, apply relevant theory and research to their work, and identify areas for further investigation.

Domain 2: Communication and interpersonal skills

1. All nurses must build partnerships and therapeutic relationships through safe, effective and non-discriminatory communication. They must take account of individual differences, capabilities and needs.

Domain 3: Nursing practice and decision-making

4. All nurses must ascertain and respond to the physical, social and psychosocial needs of people, groups and communities. They must then plan, deliver and evaluate safe, competent, person-centred care in partnership with them, paying special attention to changing health needs during different life stages, including progressive illness and death, loss and bereavement.

Domain 4: Leadership, management and team working

4. All nurses must be self-aware and recognise how their own values, principles and assumptions may affect their practice. They must maintain their own personal and professional development, learning from experience, through supervision, feedback, reflection and evaluation.

NMC Essential Skills Clusters

This chapter will address the following ESCs:

Cluster: Care, compassion and communication

3. People can trust the newly registered graduate nurse to respect them as individuals and strive to help them to preserve their dignity at all times.

continued ... •••

By the first progression point

1. Demonstrate respect for diversity and individual preference, valuing differences regardless of personal view.

By entry to the register

4. Acts professionally to ensure that personal judgements, prejudices, values, attitudes and beliefs do not compromise care.

4. People can trust the newly registered graduate nurse to engage with them and their family or carer within their cultural environments in an acceptant and antidiscriminatory manner free from harassment and exploitation.

By the first progression point

1. Demonstrates an understanding of how culture, religion, spiritual beliefs, gender and sexuality can impact on illness and disability.

By entry to the register

5. Is acceptant of differing cultural traditions, beliefs, UK legal frameworks and professional ethics when planning care with people and their families and carers.

Chapter aims

After reading this chapter you will be able to:

- consider your role in providing care for those experiencing loss, grief and bereavement;
- explain models of loss and bereavement and use these to support people, their families and carers;
- recognise differing cultural perspectives and the impact of these on nursing care of those facing loss, death and bereavement;
- support the bereaved at the end of life and care after death.

Introduction

Life seems sometimes like nothing more than a series of losses, from beginning to end. How you respond to those losses, what you make of what's left, that's the part you have to make up as you go.
(Katharine Weber, *The Music Lesson*)

As the above quote illustrates, loss and the associated grief and bereavement are about more than just death and dying. Your life is about loss, it is integral to your life and you experience loss throughout your life's journey. This may be in the form of something tangible, the loss of a family pet, leaving home, changing your job or illness. Some losses may be intangible, for example, loss of feeling safe (which may be secondary to a tangible loss) or loss of control over your body. Whilst these losses can provide a person with the opportunity to grow, this is not always the case. Take, for example, people diagnosed with motor neurone disease. Here the decline in their physical function results in a loss of control of their body and possibly their speech and affects their ability to interact with their family and friends. For the person, family and friends there is a profound sense of loss, and bereavement, long before death: loss of the life lived and loss of the life still to be lived. Indeed death might ultimately be a welcome relief. People requiring palliative and end of life care, and their carers, family and friends, will have experienced many losses, from diagnosis onwards, and will continue to do so until death.

Recognising how you respond to loss, the factors that influence this, possessing a good knowledge of the theoretical concepts of loss, grief and bereavement, recognising the impact of these and using effective strategies to support those in your care will enable you to deliver sensitive, person-centred palliative and end of life care. To support you in your ability to care for this group of people, and their carers and families, this chapter will develop your knowledge in relation to loss, grief and bereavement. In order to do this the chapter will support you in exploring your thoughts and feelings regarding loss, grief and bereavement. It will also examine the theoretical concepts of loss, grief and bereavement, recognising cultural perspectives, and will provide you with some useful strategies to support those in your care.

Exploring loss

> *Loss is defined as the state of being deprived of or being without something one has had, or a detriment or disadvantage from failure to keep, have or get. Grief is the pain and suffering experienced after loss; mourning is a period of time during which signs of grief are shown; and bereavement is the reaction to the loss of a close relationship.*
> (Humphrey and Zimpfer 2008: 3)

Loss, grief and bereavement are inextricably linked together, with each eliciting an emotional and physical response. This emotional chain commences with the loss of something, someone or some place. As such, loss can be categorised in the following ways (Humphrey and Zimpfer 2008):

- Loss of a relationship – this can be a very significant loss and may result from a break-up with a boy/girlfriend, divorce, moving to another area or death of a significant other.
- Loss of an aspect of oneself – this can be physiological, such as loss of function due to rheumatoid arthritis or loss of body part due to surgery. It can also be psychological, for example, a change in personality and sense of self following trauma, e.g., assault, or a sense of loss due to a mental health illness. In addition the loss can also be of your independence either through illness or being in prison for committing a crime.
- Loss of an external object – this can be any object that a person values and connects them to who they are; this may be a childhood toy, family heirloom or family photograph. The loss of

the object is not just in its financial value but in its sentimental significance; there is a sense of loss of self, family heritage and history.

- Developmental loss – this type of loss is a natural part of a person's growth, and is often not recognised. The very act of 'growing up' requires physical, emotional, social and psychological change and the move from carefree childhood to more responsible adolescence and adulthood. Often more visible losses can be intensified by developmental losses, e.g., a 57 year old with professional burnout may also be coping with issues of ageing.

Figure 3.1 is an example of a timeline identifying types of loss and the secondary losses experienced.

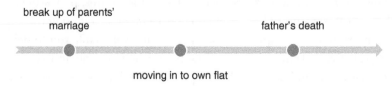

break up of parents' marriage

father's death

moving in to own flat

- Break up of parents' marriage – loss of a significant relationship, loss of an aspect of self and loss of external objects.
- Moving in to own flat – developmental loss and associated loss of significant relationships and external objects.
- Father's death – loss of significant relationship and loss of an aspect of self.

Figure 3.1: Example losses.

The above timeline allows you to see that loss is part of the fabric of life. Some losses offer you new opportunities and other losses, such as the death of a loved one, you find harder to accept.

Undertaking Activity 3.1 will support you in developing your understanding of the losses experienced by people receiving palliative and end of life care. It is important to highlight the fact that each loss is perceived differently, which means there is an element of subjectivity when we consider the ideas of loss, grief and bereavement.

Activity 3.1   *Reflection*

This exercise will assist you to explore the concept of loss, as experienced by people diagnosed and living with a life-threatening condition.

On your own or with a group of your colleagues, work through the following exercise. If you are working in a group you will need to allocate a person to read out the story.

First write down the following:

- your five most prized possessions (material things)
- your five most favourite activities

- your five most valuable body parts
- the five values that are most important to you
- the five individual people who you love the most.

Now as you read through this story, or have it read to you, cross out as many items on your list, from any category, as instructed. You must try and imagine how you might feel like while crossing off the items and what it may mean for you not having that item/person/ value any more.

It's November, the weather has turned colder, but is still dry and bright; it is the kind of morning you look forward to. You are fit and healthy and looking forward to what your life has to offer. You head out for a walk with some friends. While you are walking you start to cough and notice you are wheezing a bit.

Cross out two items.

You put it down to the colder weather, and say next time you'll wrap a scarf round your mouth. You carry on with your usual activities, however four weeks later you are still coughing; your cough is dry and irritable.

Cross out two items.

Probably a cold you think; you've been busy, some of your friends have had coughs and colds, you could probably do with resting for a couple of days. You've had mild asthma in the past, you rationalise, and carry on with your life; however something keeps niggling at the back of your mind so you make an appointment to see your doctor.

Cross out one item.

Your doctor, after examining you, refers you for a chest X-ray and takes a series of blood tests. He explains that these will be available in about a week and asks you to make another appointment to see him after this.

Cross out one item.

You visit your doctor again in a week to get your results. At this appointment your doctor tells you that there is a visible shadow on your chest X-ray and that there are changes in your bloods, specifically your liver function tests. He refers you to your local respiratory specialist team. You have a CT scan and a bronchoscopy, during which a biopsy is taken. The hospital team tell you that your results will be available in 3 days. They mention that it could be cancer, though family and friends try to reassure you that it will be OK.

Cross out three items.

Your results confirm it: you have small cell lung cancer. The CT confirms you have one lesion where your bronchus divides into 2 and further smaller lesions in your left lung. In addition both the CT and bloods confirm that this has spread to your liver. You try to remain positive and not dwell on what this might mean.

Cross out two items.

You meet with your consultant to discuss treatment options and are informed that due to the stage your cancer is at surgery is not an option. You are offered a course of four chemotherapy treatments over 3–4 months. The aim of your treatment is to shrink the size of the tumour and relieve some of your symptoms.

Cross out three items.

You start your first treatment of chemotherapy, and are encouraged as your doctor has said that the type of cancer you have responds well to chemotherapy. Unfortunately following your second treatment you develop neutropenia which requires you to be admitted to hospital for treatment and your treatment stopped. You are tired, fed up and have no appetite. You just want to be at home.

Cross out two items.

Due to your episode of neutropenia and ongoing fatigue and anorexia you find it difficult to social- ise and visit family and friends; this is important to you and provides your life with meaning and pleasure. Given this you decide not to have any further chemotherapy. Your cough and breathless- ness are getting worse, and in addition you have started to experience some chest pain. Your doctor discusses future treatment plans with you, commences you on some analgesia and suggests erlotinib (Tarceva) as a treatment to shrink your tumours. You agree to taking this.

Cross out two items.

You start to feel a bit better, your appetite returns, sort of, and your cough lessens, though you remain extremely fatigued. You try to carry on as normal though you are no longer able to manage the stairs and have your bed moved downstairs. The community health care team provides you with equipment to help you look after yourself and your family and friends help out. You attend your local hospice once a week where you enjoy having some reflexology and painting.

Cross out two items.

One morning you find it too difficult to get out of bed; you are weak and angry. Your doctor visits and, frustrated, you take it out on him. You want to stay at home but do not feel safe on your own. Your doctor suggests admission to your local hospice.

Cross out three items.

You are not sure if it is day or night; you catch a glimpse of yourself in a mirror and do not recognise yourself. You drift in and out of sleep. Friends and family visit, though you view this in slow motion; you feel removed from what is happening and wonder if this is your pain medication of if it is death approaching. You do not have the energy to ask anyone.

Cross out the last two items.

Now answer, or discuss, the following questions:

- What was it like to cross items off your list?
- What did you cross off first?
- What did you cross off last?
- Was it harder to cross off items as you went through the story?
- Did you cross off all your items or did you stop?

The above exercise is adapted from Matzo et al. (2003).

Brief answers to all activities are given at the end of the chapter, unless otherwise indicated. This activity is based on your own observations, so there is no outline answer given.

In Activity 3.1 the items you placed on your list, the order in which you crossed items off and your responses to losing your items will be unique to you. They will be influenced by many things: your age, your gender, your spiritual or religious beliefs and your cultural background. This will be the same for people diagnosed and living with a life-threatening condition; they too will have unique responses to their losses based on their individual circumstances. As individuals, with our unique perspectives on life, we can never completely *understand* how another person is feeling. Recognising your emotional responses to loss, as in Activity 3.1, will better equip you to recognise your own emotions, and the emotions of others, enabling you to empathise with those in your care. As emphasised in Activity 3.1, people living with a life-threatening condition experience loss throughout their illness, from diagnosis to end of life care. These losses can result in feelings of grief and bereavement; therefore their responses to loss may relate to known models or theories of bereavement. While this chapter focuses on loss in relation to death and dying, the principles of this can be applied to loss as it occurs in different settings and with various conditions. An understanding of the relationship between loss, grief and bereavement will support you in caring for people living with terminal illness or other illnesses that impact on their daily life. Indeed, how individuals respond to loss has been a topic of much debate and study.

Models of grief and bereavement

Not all palliative and end of life care takes place in a specialist palliative care setting. Therefore as a nurse it is likely that there will come a time when you are faced with the death of a person in your care. You are then witness to the grief, and bereavement, of the person's family, carers and friends. In some way, due to the nature of your relationship with those in your care, you share the loss with the family, carers and friends. The grief that follows loss should be recognised as a natural response to loss and there is no one way to grieve. How often have you heard someone who is bereaved say, 'I'll get over it' or 'I know I can work through this'? Alternatively you might hear a person say, 'Surely she should be over it by now' about someone who is bereaved. Grief does not just disappear; it stays with the person throughout that individual's life.

Your role is to provide support that allows the bereaved person to find a place for his or her grief while enabling the person to carry on *living*. Death and dying can provoke strong emotional responses in us (see Chapter 1). Being self-aware, and recognising and managing the emotions you experience in relation to loss, grief and bereavement will enable you to develop positive therapeutic relationships with those in your care (see Nicol 2015).

Over the past century or so many models and theories have attempted to explain and rationalise people's experiences of grief in response to a significant loss and subsequent change in their life. These models have discussed grief and bereavement from a variety of perspectives, such as the stages of grief, the process of grief and attachment and loss. Understanding these models will provide you with knowledge of the broad theoretical concepts. Applying these to those in your care will assist you to support those who are bereaved. When applying these models to people in your care, you should be aware of the influence their values, beliefs and culture have on them and how these shape their experience of grief and bereavement. Doing this will enable you to deliver person-centred culturally sensitive care that recognises and celebrates the diverse population in the UK. Chapter 4 discusses aspects of culture and caring in a multicultural way. There is not scope in this book to discuss all models and theories; further reading is mentioned at the end of the chapter. However, it is pertinent that we discuss the seminal works and some of the more recent models and theories.

Sigmund Freud: *Mourning and Melancholia*

Sigmund Freud, in his seminal work *Mourning and Melancholia* (1917), was perhaps the first person to put forward an explanation of grief and bereavement. Written against the backdrop of the First World War, Freud recognised the attachment people had to the deceased and that in grief people who are bereaved give up not only the deceased but also a part of themselves. In his discussions Freud stated the requirement for the bereaved to disengage from what has been lost, withdraw energy, and subsequently invest this energy in new attachments. In doing this he recognised the many layers of attachment and the secondary losses that are present. This suggestion by Freud would mean that the bereaved may not continue with their life until they have successfully detached themselves emotionally from the deceased. This has attracted criticism as most people believe they can carry on with their life without completely detaching themselves from the deceased. The important thing to say is that people learn to manage their emotions and now and again can put them to one side (compartmentalise them) while concentrating on the here and now of life.

Kübler-Ross: *On Death and Dying*

Elisabeth Kübler-Ross's work *On Death and Dying* (1973) is perhaps the most widely recognised work in the area of loss, grief and bereavement. Her study was based on the belief that most people feared dying, *not* death, with people believing it to be a lonely, impersonal experience. Her aim was to understand this process better and so support those who are dying in coming to terms with their own mortality. Kübler-Ross interviewed over 200 people who were dying, encouraging them to discuss their thoughts and feelings about their own dying and death. From these interviews she identified five stages people who are dying experience: denial, anger, bargaining, depression and acceptance. The stages are seen as coping mechanisms, defence strategies or ways of maintaining hope that can overlap or exist at the same time and are human responses to dying. Therefore, it should be recognised that those who are dying may not experience all of these stages or experience them in that order.

Activity 3.2   *Critical thinking*

Take the time to consider some of the issues that you might be faced with when applying Kübler-Ross's work to those who are facing loss.

In Activity 3.2 you might have identified that you may 'expect' people to grieve in a particular way or order and that this could impact on the care you provide. It is ideas like these that have led to criticism of Kübler-Ross's theory; these include the research methodology used (Kastenbaum 2011). Gathering information from different sources, e.g., patient diaries, would have added to the rigour of the study. Additionally the stages could be viewed as prescriptive rather than descriptive, with individuals feeling that they have to move from one stage to the next and becoming concerned when they do not or can not. Perhaps most importantly Kübler-Ross's theory could be seen as distilling a person's life down to a series of stages that fail to recognise the individuality of the person, and that they are still living. These are all important factors to consider when delivering holistic person-centred palliative and end of life care. Despite these more recent critisims it should be remembered that Kübler-Ross spoke up about death and dying at a time when they were taboo subjects and provided a voice for those who felt isolated, providing them with an opportunity to teach others about their experience.

Klass, Silverman and Nickman: *Continuing Bonds*

The model proposed by Klass et al. (1996) called into question previous perceptions that stated grief was something to work through and a detachment from the deceased needed to be made, in other words to 'break the bonds' with the deceased. Klass et al. (1996) stated that bereavement should be considered as a cognitive and emotional process that takes place in the context of a person's life, of which the deceased person is part. Their work proposed that maintaining bonds with the deceased was normal in mourning and could contribute to successful adaptation of the bereavement. An example of this could be that the bereaved person takes into consideration the viewpoint of the deceased when making decisions, using the deceased as a guide. This approach could have a positive effect on the bereaved through finding positive meaning in life and increased emotional resilience. It should be recognised however that in some instances continuing bonds could be harmful. There is a link between externalising continuing bonds, e.g., hearing the deceased's voice, talking about them in the present tense and violent loss (or loss where the bereaved was very emotionally dependent on the deceased). Here research has shown that there is a relationship between this type of continuing bond and complicated grief, that could indicate that the loss has not been integrated (Field and Filanosky 2009). On the whole though maintaining a continuing bond with the deceased preserves memories. Goodhead (2010) analysed memorials to deceased loved ones on the St Christopher's Hospice 'Tree of Life'. His analysis found that continuing bonds, declaring an ongoing loving relationship between the bereaved and deceased, featured in up to 69.6 per cent of the memorials written.

Stroebe and Schut: the Dual Process Model

The Dual Process Model introduced new thinking in relation to loss, grief and bereavement. Rather than focusing solely on 'grief work', it emphasised the role that other coping strategies play in helping the bereaved (Stroebe and Schut 1999). Stroebe and Schut explain that grieving is a dynamic process where the bereaved oscillate between different coping behaviours (everyday life experiences) termed 'loss orientation' and 'restoration orientation'. Loss orientation focuses on the loss of the person who has died and includes grief work, e.g., talking about the loss, crying. Restoration orientation incorporates addressing the additional losses faced by the bereaved, such as returning to work or managing household finances. This oscillation allows the bereaved person to take time off from the pain of grief, which can be overwhelming, enabling the bereaved to cope with day-to-day life and the changes in it.

The Dual Process Model emphasises that both loss orientation and restoration orientation are necessary to allow the bereaved to adjust to their new future. However the authors recognise that the emphasis on loss orientation and restoration orientation will vary from person to person depending on the circumstances of the death and the personality, gender, age and cultural background of the bereaved. Stroebe and Schut state that this model can also be used to identify complicated or unresolved grief, allowing appropriate therapeutic interventions to be put in place. This can be used to support bereavement counselling by identifying which part of the model the person spends most of their time in. Strategies can then be implemented to support the person to manage grief and bereavement more positively.

Applying the models to your care

Gaining knowledge and developing an understanding of these models will assist you to identify where a person is in his or her grief. Read through the case study below and consider which models of loss, grief and bereavement are relevant.

Case study

Paul's adult son Matt (himself a father) had type 1 diabetes, Paul had known that poor management of his diabetes would affect Matt's life expectancy but Paul had not expected him to die quite so soon. Due to diabetic peripheral neuropathy Paul had anticipated that Matt may require an amputation, but he had not considered Matt would have a catastrophic subarachnoid haemorrahge (SAH). Immediately following Matt's SAH, despite the fact he was in an induced coma, Paul remained optimistic: his son's condition would improve, they were taking one day at a time. This was in contrast to Sarah, Paul's wife, who stated early on that she did not feel Matt would survive. Ten days following his SAH Matt was declared 'brain dead' and the decision was taken to switch off his life support. Paul, Sarah and their surviving children found this a difficult decision to make. Paul, in particular, delayed the decision twice before it took place.

After Matt's life support was switched off Paul 'took charge'; it was his responsibility to arrange the funeral, clear out his son's flat and inform his friends. He was a practical person and taking on this provided him with a purpose. Sarah, on the other hand, was much more willing to talk about Matt and what had happened. She found it frustrating that Paul would not talk about Matt, apart from in a practical sense: 'Which type of coffin do you think Matt would have liked?' The day of the funeral arrived and Paul was in charge, telling people which car they were to be in, telling family and friends where to sit at the crematorium. At the 'wake' following the funeral Paul spent his time chatting to Matt's friends, hearing stories about his son and reminiscing with his friends.

A few months after Matt's death Paul still did not speak about Matt. His surviving children were concerned and worried that he was not 'coping' but were unsure how to approach this with him as any suggestion was met negatively. Sarah tried to support both her children and husband, encouraging each to see the other's point of view, but in the end this only aggravated things. Unspoken, the decision was made to leave Paul to 'work it out himself'. Paul's main source of comfort was Lizzy, Matt's youngest daughter. They became inseparable: they went for walks together, Paul helped Lizzy with her school work and they spoke about Matt. Paul liked Lizzy's open and honest approach to Matt's death – it was refreshing.

Matt's family found the first year hard: birthdays, anniversaries and family holidays came and went. Gradually Paul began to open up and rebuild his relationships with his wife and children, though he still maintained a strong bond with Lizzy. His own health scare 16 months after Matt's death re-emphasised to him the fragility of life and the importance of family and friends.

It is evident in the case study that a number of models of loss, grief and bereavement are applicable to Paul and his family. In the early days Paul has feelings of denial about Matt's situation, believing that Matt's condition will improve, whereas Sarah, his wife, is more accepting. Here you could identify Paul and Sarah as experiencing different stages of the stages of dying, as discussed by Kübler-Ross (1973). It is also possible to identify elements of the Dual Process Model (Stroebe and Schut 1999), with Paul focusing on restoration orientation by helping her to organise Matt's funeral and Sarah focusing on loss orientation in her desire to talk about her son. When we consider Klass et al.'s (1996) continuing bonds it can be seen that this is also evident in Paul's bereavement. Through spending time with Lizzy, and getting to know her better, Paul has chosen to maintain a significant bond with Matt.

Activity 3.3   *Reflection*

Using the information above, reflect back on your previous practice or placement experience. Which models of loss and bereavement have you seen displayed in people, carers, family or staff? You may find it helpful to read the article by Buglass (2010) to develop your understanding of these models. The full reference for this article is listed in the further reading section at the end of this chapter.

As this activity is based on your own observations, there is no outline answer at the end of this chapter.

Both the case study above and Activity 3.3 will have enabled you to explore the various responses people have when faced with the death of a loved one. Having a good understanding of the models and how they apply to your clinical practice will assist you in recognising how people who are bereaved respond. It will also enable you to discuss loss, grief and bereavement with bereaved people, reassuring them that their response is natural.

It is important that you understand that you may end up using different aspects from different models and use them together to help support the person and the bereaved. With practice you will develop skills to select the most useful 'bits' from a range of different models for your own use. For example, where there is denial you may allow more time for the bereaved to come to terms with their loss. And where there is anger, you may want to acknowledge it and then empathise as a starting point in helping the bereaved. As part of the case study and Activity 3.3 you may also have identified anticipatory grief, for example in the case study where Paul recognises that Matt's type 1 diabetes may affect his life expectancy. Indeed you may also have identified this when participating in Activity 3.1 as you faced anticipating losing what is important to you.

Anticipatory grief

Anticipatory grief may be present from point of diagnosis on, not only for the person diagnosed but for their family and carers. This is particularly poignant for the family and carers of people with dementia as they anticipate the gradual loss of their loved one's personality. Given the increase in the number of people being diagnosed with dementia (current global numbers are 47.5 million with projections that this will rise to 75.6 million by 2030 (Alzheimer's Disease International 2015)), there is growing interest in anticipatory grief and dementia with research being undertaken to understand this more fully.

Research summary: anticipatory grief and dementia

In 2012 Chan et al. published a systematic review exploring the grief reactions, both before (anticipatory) and after death, of family carers looking after a person with dementia. Their review focused on: characteristics, prevalence, predictors and associations of anticipatory and post-death grief in dementia. Their search resulted in a total of 31 papers being included in their review. Chan et al. (2012) used recognised assessment tools with which to assess the quality of the studies. Each study was scored out of 8 and independently reviewed by two of the authors; where inconsistencies appeared another reviewer was involved to moderate. This ensured triangulation of data and contributed to reducing potential bias. In relation to anticipatory grief their findings can be summarised as follows:

- Characteristics – grief and loss. The review identified several high quality studies that identified feelings of ambiguity about the future, sadness and the loss of intimacy and personal freedom. The relationship to the person with dementia was also significant with adult children and spouses responding in different ways. Adult children displayed denial (early dementia) and anger/frustration (moderate dementia), whereas the spouse exhibited acceptance (early dementia) and empathy (moderate dementia), though it was also identified that as the person's dementia progressed, the family/carer displayed increasing grief reactions. In severe dementia both the adult children and spouse accepted institutionalisation with sadness and relief from the burden of caring (respectively). However Chan et al. note that institutionalisation can also increase feelings of guilt and failure.
- Prevalence – this was found to range between 47 per cent and 71 per cent, though it was recognised by Chan et al. that there were no high quality studies exploring prevalence, so these results should be treated with caution.
- Predictors and associations – all of the areas discussed in this theme were found in high quality research studies. The emotional and mental health of the carer was identified as being associated with anticipatory grief, with a correlation between anticipatory grief and depression and poor emotional health. Other factors identified include: the burden being placed on the carer, difficulties arising over any language barrier, e.g., non-English speaker in an English-speaking country, and reduced satisfaction with the care received.

Chan et al. recognise the limitations of their review; some of the studies reviewed used small sample sizes and were from the United States, therefore results may not be generalisable. In addition some studies did not provide a clear definition of grief, meaning there could be ambiguity in some of the features displayed, e.g., carer anxiety. However this is the first study to use a systematic review to explore this area and the results can be used to inform further research.

It is recognised that Chan et al. (2012) explored both anticipatory and post-death grief, but for the purposes of this chapter only the results for anticipatory grief have been included.

You can use the themes identified in Chan et al.'s (2012) work to support the care you provide to the family and carers of people with dementia. Recognising the feelings of loss and grief experienced by carers, how they change as the person's dementia progresses and increasing your understanding of this will also ensure that you are aware of the contributing factors that could increase a person's anticipatory grief, e.g., depression. This will, in turn, allow you to put in place strategies to support the carers and minimise the likelihood of adverse grief reactions following the death of the person with dementia.

Case study

My dad was diagnosed with Alzheimer's disease three years ago when he was only 52 years old. I was 19, and my sister was 15. The first time we knew anything was wrong was when dad phoned mum saying that he could not remember how to get home; he had been out on a business appointment (he is a freelance graphic designer), and mum and I had to go and drive him home. It was only after this that mum and dad told us about dad's diagnosis. None of us could believe it; dementia was something that happened to old people not young, healthy people like my dad. We were all in a state of shock; my sister refused to believe it, my brother and I felt incredibly frustrated and scared about how dad's condition might progress. Mum seemed remarkably accepting of the situation, but then she had known dad's diagnosis for about six months, and tried to focus on the positives.

Dad was determined to keep working, though due to his ability to get lost so easily when driving, mum became his unofficial chauffeur! She was, and still is amazing, she could see how important working was for dad and she was determined to support him to do this for as long as possible. It really felt like mum understood how dad was feeling. Roles in the family changed: mum took over managing household finances, my sister and I tried to get on better with each other so there was less arguing and shouting. We realised how important it was for dad to feel secure and arguing only made him feel anxious.

As dad's condition progressed his behavior began to change, his moods became unpredictable and he would become angry very quickly. He forgot which cupboard things were in and was forever asking questions. My sister found this difficult to deal with; she didn't understand why he would get angry and became frustrated with dad when he forgot things, walking away and refusing to help him. She stopped inviting friends round and began to spend most of her time out of the house at her best friend's. At this time I remember feeling very sad, thinking how scared I would feel if it was me. I put notices on the kitchen cupboards with pictures of what was on each shelf. The first time I did this dad took them down, and I remember him saying to me 'I'm not stupid, don't treat me like a child'. This hurt me deeply, but I could see his point of view.

Perhaps the most surprising thing was how my sister's attitude towards dad changed. One day instead of walking away when dad was angry she put on some of his favourite music. The change in dad was almost immediate – he calmed down and started singing along and my sister joined in! When I asked her about it later she told me she had read about research into the role music has in calming people who have dementia. Knowing this and seeing the effects has changed how we think about managing some of dad's symptoms and has enabled us all to participate in caring for him. We all know things are going to get worse, and we know as dad's condition deteriorates our relationships with him will change. Therefore we focus on the here and now, spending as much time doing the things dad wants to do.

Activity 3.4   *Evidence-based practice and research*

Reading the case study and the research summary above, consider anticipatory grief as it is affecting the family. What coping mechanisms are they using to manage their grief?

Completing Activity 3.4 will have enabled you to see how the topics discussed so far in this chapter all interlink: the ongoing nature of loss that is felt from the point of diagnosis onwards, the anticipation of the grief to come as losses are adjusted to and managed, the pre- and post-bereavement and how models can be used to identify this in people's actions and behaviour. Recognising the individual nature of loss and how it can be expressed will support you to provide person-centred care for the person receiving palliative and end of life care, their family and carers. Increasing your awareness of how you respond to loss, grief and bereavement, and what strategies you use to cope will increase your own emotional resilience and ability to care in emotionally challenging situations.

Religious considerations in loss, grief and bereavement

The previous discussions in this chapter have shown that people who are dying have their sense of 'self' and what is important to them challenged. Promoting a sense of uniqueness, and assisting a person to find meaning in their life and to integrate that meaning, can support a person to prepare for their death. Recognising this spiritual aspect of a person can also alleviate a person's anxiety about death and may include specific religious practices (Kisvetrova et al. 2013). To support this, the National Institute for Health and Care Excellence's quality standards for end of life care for adults (NICE 2013) recognise the need for a person's religion to be addressed as part of holistic care at end of life:

- Standard 6: people approaching the end of life are offered spiritual and religious support appropriate to their needs and preferences;
- Standard 12: the body of a person who has died is cared for in a culturally sensitive and dignified manner. In addition, standard 12 should recognise that people who are dying and who have died should be cared for in accordance with their religious teachings.

One thing is certain: whatever a person's spiritual and/or religious orientation they will be touched by death in a way that is unique to them. Therefore, how they grieve and mourn will be strongly influenced by their religious orientation, with most religions having developed rituals related to grief and mourning (Rosenblatt 2015). It is recognised that the religious profile of the UK is changing. An increasing number of people state secular views, 15.5 per cent of the population in 2001 and 25 per cent in 2011, and the number of people stating Christianity as their religion is falling, from 71.6 per cent in 2001 to 59 per cent in 2011. In contrast most minority religions have seen an increase in numbers with the number of people stating Islam as their religion increasing by over 1 million (Office for National Statistics 2012). You need to respond to this more religiously diverse demographic by providing person-centred care that is sensitive to people's religious needs. This section only focuses on religious aspects: you can read more about cultural care in Chapter 4.

Case study

Ali is 65 years old and has been living with chronic kidney disease since he was 25. He is a devout Muslim and lives with his wife Nabila. They have three children: two daughters, Nyla and Sanna, and a son, Tariq. Ali's children and their families all live close by and are very supportive. Ali's faith is very important to him and it has helped to keep him strong throughout his life.

Recently Ali has been told that his second kidney transplant is failing and, following a conversation with his family, Ali has decided not to have any more dialysis. Ali and his family know that by refusing further dialysis his condition will deteriorate and he will eventually die. Ali has accepted this, but is worried about the impact of this on his family. Ali has stated that he would like to remain in his own home, and if possible die there, and this is an arrangement all his family are in agreement with.

For Muslims, illness and disease may be regarded as a test from Allah. Therefore both the person who is ill and their family may take comfort and find spiritual healing in reciting the Qur'an (Taheri 2008). Muslims believe that their death is preordained: *no soul can die save with the permission of Allah* (3:145). Death is not the cessation of this life; the person's spirit is eternal and lives on. For many Muslims, health and illness are part of the continuum of being, with prayer providing salvation in both health and sickness. One important point to emphasise is that this may be different to how you or your family approach death and dying. When caring for a person with differing values and beliefs, maybe like Ali, it is crucial that you remind yourself to respect their preferences and wishes, even if you do not agree with them.

Activity 3.5   *Evidence-based practice and research*

Two days ago Ali's condition deteriorated quite quickly. The Primary Care Team recognised that Ali was entering the terminal stages of life and discussed this with his family. Ali's family decided that they would care for him at home with support from the District Nursing Team. You are working with the District Nurse (DN) and visit Ali and his family twice a day to offer support.

Task 1

In order to respect Ali's and his family's Islamic faith, what care do you need to take into consideration during his final days?

One afternoon, whilst visiting another patient, the DN you are working with receives a phone call from Ali's son. He says his dad's condition is worsening; his breathing is becoming more laboured. The DN explains to Tariq that she will be with them as soon as she can. When you arrive at Ali's house you are met by his son, who says his dad has died.

Task 2

In order to respect Ali's and his family's Islamic faith, what do you need to take into consideration now that he has died?

To help you answer these questions use the following reference:

Alladin, W. (2015) The Islamic way of death and dying, in Murray Parkes, C., Laungani, P. and Young, B. (eds) *Death and Bereavement Across Cultures*. 2nd edn. Hove: Routledge, 111–132.

Activity 3.5 has focused on the religious aspects of Ali's care before and after death. As well as recognising these, it is important that you utilise effective communication skills and demonstrate non-judgemental care, e.g., active listening, reflecting and accepting the family's thoughts and feelings. Following Ali's death the family will adhere to a period of mourning; this is generally for three days and is known as *hidad*. It is likely that the women and men will mourn separately. During this period of mourning the Qur'an will be recited. During *hidad* it is customary for friends and family to visit the bereaved and offer their condolences. Ali's family will not prepare any food; this will be prepared by their friends, relatives and other members of their community. Nabila, Ali's widow, will observe a longer period of mourning (*iddah*) which lasts for four months and ten days.

This case study and activity focus specifically on Ali and his individual needs. The knowledge you have gained from reading this chapter will enable you to apply these principles to your nursing practice in palliative and end of life care, taking into consideration people's religious, spiritual and other preferences.

Care after death

For many the concept of a 'good death' includes not just the care given up to the time of death but also the care given to the deceased after death (Pattison 2008). It is know that sensitive care after death can support families to make sense of what is happening and facilitate grieving and should be based on the families' needs and wishes (Berry and Griffe 2015), though it is recognised that you should follow any national and local guidelines, to ensure safe practice. The care given after death encompasses what has, in nursing, been traditionally referred to as 'last offices'. The term 'last offices' not only relates to nursing's military and religious roots but also to the Christian sacrament of 'last rites' (Quested and Rudge 2003).

Research by Martin and Bristowe (2015) into the experiences of nurses carrying out care after death identified three overlapping themes: a demonstration of respect and support, a time of transition and a learning and coping challenge. Participants described trying to see the person and where they were through the eyes of their family. This was evidenced by care they took when carrying out care after death, talking to the person, making them look clean and tidy, dressing them in their own clothes and in making the room peaceful, creating a lasting peaceful image of the person. In addition participants recognised the significance of performing care after death in relation to their own coping and viewed it as an opportunity to 'close the chapter' and progress to caring for their next patient.

Activity 3.6   *Reflection*

Using a model of reflection, e.g., Gibbs (1988), and the following questions as prompts, reflect back on a situation where you have performed care after death. If you have not performed care after death yourself, discuss these questions with your mentor/registered nurse:

- If appropriate, how were cultural and religious practices addressed/maintained during care after death?
- How were the privacy and dignity of the deceased maintained?
- Was there any aspect of performing care after death that you found particularly difficult? If yes, then why was this?
- Were there any aspects of performing care after death that you found particularly comforting? If yes, what were they?
- How did you demonstrate support for the bereaved?

Using a model of reflection will assist you to structure your reflection, ensuring that you stay focused on a specific topic. Using the questions listed will further increase your level of analysis of the situation, and this will develop your ability to analyse critically your own practice and that of colleagues.

As this activity is based on your own observations, there is no outline answer at the end of this chapter.

As you can see from Activity 3.5, when performing care after death, as well as caring for the deceased and the bereaved, it is important that you take care of yourself. To be able to perform care after death in a positive way you need to possess an understanding of the skills and emotional resilience you require to enable you to carry out this act (Nyatanga and de Vocht 2009).

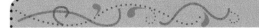

Chapter summary

This chapter has provided you with an overview of loss, grief and bereavement and its application to holistic care in palliative and end of life care. The concept of loss has been explored and models of grief and bereavement have been discussed and applied to a case scenario. This approach will support you in recognising the individuality of bereavement and how a person's grief changes over time and the importance of maintaining bonds with the deceased. Recognising anticipatory grief and its role in loss, grief and bereavement in relation to caring for people with dementia has been explored and related to nursing practice. The importance of respecting and honouring a person's religious requirements at end of life has been discussed. The effect of sensitive care after death on the bereaved, and you as a nurse, has been recognised.

Activities: brief outline answers

Activity 3.2: Critical thinking

Having a fixed, linear idea of how a person will grieve could impact negatively on the type of post-bereavement care you provide. For example, when a bereaved person has accepted the death of the loved one early in the grieving process, this could be misinterpreted as complicated grief, with the offer of bereavement counselling seen as inappropriate. This could result in the bereaved person feeling that you are not listening to his or her needs, resulting in a loss of trust and a breakdown in the therapeutic relationship. This could subsequently prevent the bereaved person from seeking support from you in the future, if necessary.

Activity 3.4: Evidence-based practice and research

Each member of the family responds in different ways; perhaps the person affected most visibly was the younger daughter who displayed very clearly denial and frustration in the early days of her dad's diagnosis. She managed this by removing herself from the family, both emotionally and physically. This could be viewed as negative, however it may have been giving her the time and space needed to come to terms with her dad's diagnosis. Towards the end of the case study she takes a much more positive approach, which impacts on all the family. Perhaps her initial denial meant that she took the time to find out about Alzheimer's and how to manage it.

The mum took on a more supportive role earlier on; she seemed to emphathise very early on with how her husband might be feeling and her focus was on supporting him to 'live well'. This positive approach may help to maintain her mental and emotional health as her husband's condition deteriorates as she can be confident that she did all she could to maintain his sense of self. There are also parallels with the Dual Process Model and restoration orientation, taking on the role of managing the family finances.

Through feeling frustrated early on the older daughter seems to have taken quite a practical approach to helping her dad, though this was not always welcome. However, this does not put her off; she tries an alternative way which is successful. This problem solving approach will be key as her dad's condition deteriorates and more challenges are faced.

Activity 3.5: Evidence-based practice and research

Task 1

- Support Ali's family to ensure that the local imam is available.
- It is important, where possible, that the soles of Ali's feet face the Qiblah in Mecca (direction in the UK south-east); therefore Ali's bed should be moved to allow this to happen. If this is not possible, then it is permissible for Ali's face to be turned to the direction of the Qiblah.
- Friends and relatives should be allowed to gather round Ali.

- Privacy should be allowed as family members may wish to recite prayers; this will include the Declaration of Faith (Shahada) which is regarded as a blessed act and the person's last prayer. If Ali is not able to say this himself then it will be said by a family member and whispered gently over Ali's face.

Task 2

- Once the death has been verified, Ali's body should be prepared in accordance with the wishes of his family.
- Ali's body should be treated in a gentle and dignified manner.
- If at all possible, only people of the same sex as the deceased should touch the body; therefore only males should touch Ali (where practical).
- After his death Ali's body should not be touched by a non-Muslim. Therefore it would be appropriate to ask permission first from the family and to wear gloves.
- Ali should not be left with his feet facing the Qiblah. Instead his body should be positioned to allow his face to be turned to the right and face the Qiblah.
- Ali's eyes should be closed and his body straightened out. This is done by flexing and straightening the elbows, shoulders, knees and hips, in the belief that it will prevent Ali's body from stiffening.
- Any excess fluid, blood or excrement can be cleaned from Ali's body, though his nails should not be cut. Ritual cleansing will be carried out as soon as possible by a male Muslim.
- Ali's body should remain covered at all times.
- Ensure that all documentation is completed in a timely manner. This reduces the likelihood of any delay in the funeral taking place; burials take place within 24 hours.

Further reading

Buglass, E. (2010) Grief and bereavement theories. *Nursing Standard*, 24 (41): 44–47.

This article provides a review of the most well-known bereavement models.

Pattison, N. (2008) Care of patients who have died. *Nursing Standard*, 22 (28): 42–48.

This article outlines the steps involved in preparing the deceased after death, including religious and legal considerations, and aftercare for the family.

Useful websites

www.dyingmatters.org

This is the website for the Dying Matters coalition; their aim is to raise awareness of, and change attitudes towards, death, dying and bereavement. Their site contains useful resources for both health care professionals and those living with dying, on relevant topics relating to death and dying.

www.endoflifecare-intelligence.org.uk/home

This is the website for the National End of Life Care Programme. The aim of this programme is to improve end of life care for adults in England. However there is information on this site that is applicable to all people who are receiving palliative and end of life care.

Chapter 4
Understanding cultural issues in palliative and end of life care

Brian Nyatanga

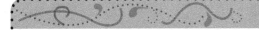

NMC Standards for Pre-registration Nursing Education

This chapter will address the following competencies:

Domain 1: Professional values

2. All nurses must practise in a holistic, non-judgemental, caring and sensitive manner that avoids assumptions; supports social inclusion; recognises and respects individual choice; and acknowledges diversity. Where necessary, they must challenge inequality, discrimination and exclusion from access to care.

Domain 2: Communication and interpersonal skills

1. All nurses must build partnerships and therapeutic relationships through safe, effective and non-discriminatory communication. They must take account of individual differences, capabilities and needs.

NMC Essential Skills Clusters

This chapter will address the following ESCs:

Cluster: Care, compassion and communication

3. People can trust a newly qualified graduate nurse to respect them as individuals and strive to help them preserve their dignity at all times.

First progression point

1. Demonstrates respect for diversity and individual preference, valuing differences, regardless of personal view

Entry to the register

4. Acts professionally to ensure that personal judgements, prejudices, values, attitudes and beliefs do not compromise care

4. People can trust a newly qualified graduate nurse to engage with them and their family or carers within their cultural environments in an acceptant and anti-discriminatory manner free from harassment and exploitation.

continued …

First progression point

1. Demonstrates an understanding of how culture, religion, spiritual beliefs, gender and sexuality can impact on illness and disability.

Entry to the register

5. Is acceptant of differing cultural traditions, beliefs, UK legal frameworks and professional ethics when planning care with people and their families and carers.
6. Acts autonomously and proactively in promoting care environments that are culturally sensitive and free from discrimination, harassment and exploitation.

Chapter aims

After reading this chapter you will be able to:

*   discuss the idea of culture and how it is transmitted from one generation to the next;
*   explore possible modifications to culture as a result of current changes in the world with particular focus on Brexit in the UK;
*   explore cultural differences and associated issues of immigration when caring for people receiving palliative and end of life care;
*   explore the idea of multicultural society and the need for health care professionals to be culturally competent in their care for dying patients;
*   discuss what type of knowledge and skills health care professionals need to become culturally competent in caring for diverse patient groups.

Introduction

Cultural differences do not exist to cause conflict; instead they are a way of enhancing our unity, exploring different realities and therefore increase our power of knowledge.
(Luca Carvana)

The power of knowledge makes a difference in how we perceive the world, other countries, their leaders, our own society, health care professionals and patients we care for. Luca Carvana's quote above distances us from the ever growing misconception and rhetoric that cultural difference equates to hatred, conflict, war and even killings of one man by another, one ethnic group by another. The truth is that to be different is not the issue here; it is our lack of understanding of difference that is the real problem. What compounds the problem is how we try and resolve differences. Some choose to separate or isolate themselves from those who are different, some think building walls between nations is the answer, and others resort to hate, terror, destruction and killings of those that are different. Such strategies seem short-sighted, self-centred and serve no realistic purpose in a continually growing and changing world. For the world at large and palliative care professionals in particular, what is needed is to appreciate the different backgrounds, identities and preferences of other people. Caring in a multicultural society like the UK needs awareness of culture, cultural differences and those central rituals that not only distinguish groups but guide and justify their existence. This chapter discusses the idea of culture and cultural competence in palliative care settings. It also considers the impact of the referendum result in June 2016 for the UK to leave the European Union (Brexit). This appears to have been, at least in part, an outcome of many people in the UK being uncomfortable with the increasing cultural and ethnic diversity resulting from the European Union policy of free movement of people between member states. Later the same year saw the election of the Republican Donald Trump as President of the United States, taking office in January 2017. Trump's election rhetoric included a number of divisive messages about the poor, disabled, women and LGBTQ communities but two position statements stand out:

- The banning of Muslims from entering the USA and
- The building of a wall between the USA and Mexico.

There are other global examples suggestive of cultural intolerance among people but the two examples given above suffice to make the point about the changing nature of cultural relationships around the world. The implication of these changes for palliative care is the focus for this chapter, along with suggestions of how to still achieve cultural competence for the dying patient and their family.

In palliative care, attending to and being aware of cultural differences is one of the central pillars of unique individualised care you provide at the end of life. It is quite possible that the dying patients in your care may experience similar diagnoses and symptoms, but each of them may attach a different meaning to these. These meanings will be formed by individuals' character, life experiences and cultural background and expectations. Therefore, if you and other health care professionals are to provide patient-centred care, you will need to recognise such individual and cultural differences. Living, as we now do, in a multicultural Britain (and indeed a multicultural world), we need to become *culturally competent*. As a first step towards achieving this, let us consider what culture is and what it means for different people.

Understanding culture

The word *culture* is often used in different ways and contexts, and at times is used to refer to race, skin colour and nationality. The term is also used in relation to work practices such as the 'culture of care' in hospices or care homes, or in wider fields – for example, 'the culture of people trafficking', the 'culture of using performance-enhancing drugs' in sport. These examples show that 'culture' as a term is not easy to define or understand, and that it may not have a universal definition or meaning. Indeed, you may have a different understanding of the term. Activity 4.1 gives you an opportunity to explore your own understanding of culture.

In Activity 4.1 you may have sought to describe culture from a social perspective, which tends to be a common theme when writing on the subject. From this social view, culture is considered to be what governs a group of people in how they live their lives: the attitudes, values and beliefs those people hold and share *as a group*. It is important to say you cannot actually see the beliefs and values people hold. This is where the behaviour of people towards something can 'tell' you about their beliefs, attitudes and subsequently their culture. For example, you would not be able to tell by looking at a person whether he or she was Christian, vegetarian or racist unless you saw them at church or eating their meals, or discriminating against someone based on race. These behaviours alone may not be sufficient to confirm what the person holds inside them (beliefs and values), therefore, it is safer to infer that what we see in behaviour is a reflection of their beliefs and values. However, we often find that people with similar beliefs and values *may* also share physical aspects such as skin colour, living space and geographical backgrounds. For example, people living in the same region may share similar values and beliefs about marriage, whereas student nurses working together may end up sharing some values about how to care for dying patients with compassion. You may want to suggest that the nursing students would have similar professional cultural values that guide their practice. The commonly used social definition talks about culture being *a set of attitudes, values and beliefs shared by a group of people and [that] tend to govern their behaviour in society* (Matsumoto and Juang 2012). However, earlier writers using an anthropological lens saw 'culture' as referring to *patterns explicit and implicit of and for behaviour acquired and transmitted by symbols, language and rituals* (Kroeber and Kluckholm 1952). (Anthropology is the study of societies, cultures and human origins.)

The first part of your activity can be explained by acknowledging that people are different; we all see and believe in different ways of living our lives. Those differences may also be witnessed when we consider culture and what it means to different people. So many of our responses and behaviours as we go through life are shaped by the views we hold about the world and culture is an integral part of this. For some, past experience can influence their view of culture whereas others may find events in the present changing their views. For example, events of summer 2016 in the UK suggest a shift in attitudes towards multiculturalism with an increase in immigration being seen (wrongly) as the cause of problems such as housing shortages, social unrest and lack of funding for the NHS.

Categories of culture

The above description falls under the *normative* category of culture. As far back as 1992, Berry and others came up with different categories of culture (Table 4.1) as a way of showing some of the fine difference between the categories. The fact that there have not been any recent attempts to provide different categories suggests that most researchers accept this categorisation of culture.

If you look closely at Table 4.1, you will see that the categories tend to overlap. This shows how culture is intertwined into different aspects of people's ways of life.

Type of culture	Description	Comment
Descriptive	Focuses on different activities or behaviours associated with a culture	Used to enhance understanding
Historical	Refers to the heritage and traditions associated with a group of people	Similar to genetic
Normative	Focuses on rules and norms associated with a culture	Commonly used with definitions
Psychological	Focuses on learning and problem solving in order to strengthen a culture	Rarely discussed, and poorly understood
Structural	Focuses on societal and organisational structures of a cultural group	Often implied in the discussion
Genetic	Focuses on origins of a culture	Similar to historical

Table 4.1: Categories of culture, based on Berry et al. (1992)

You may be wondering how these characteristics differ from religion, at least where people of faith are concerned. Thinking in this way shows that you are beginning to grasp the finer points about culture and that they may sometimes have strong connections with organised religion. However, the simple answer is that culture and religion are different.

Activity 4.2   *Reflection*

Take some time to reflect on what you already know about religion, and write down how religion differs from culture.

As the answers to this activity will be based on your own reflections, no outline answer is given at the end of the chapter. However, a discussion of some of the issues involved is below.

You might have found Activity 4.2 quite difficult as it can be challenging to try and separate these two entities. The way some people live can be influenced by both culture and religion.

Both culture and religion are underpinned by beliefs and values that hold and guide the way people live their lives. You can begin to separate these two if you consider what people do to fulfil their cultural and religious needs. Religious people would probably pray, go to a place of worship or attend gatherings to share thoughts and prayers. Another way of separating these two is when we include people who do not have a religion (faith) to guide their lives. For example, atheists (people who do not believe in God) or those without any faith whatsoever, or even those who do not know what they believe (agnostics) still have a culture. However, the way in which they go about fulfilling their cultural needs would be through different ritualistic practices – such as visiting the sea every year – rather than by going to church, temple or mosque, all of which are equally valid and demonstrate the depth and breadth of cultural and religious practices.

Some understanding of culture is necessary if you are to understand yourself and others (in terms of beliefs and values) and your place in a changing world. It is also helpful for identifying the sort of world we would like to live in, and how this aspiration can be carried through or passed down to younger generations. The world continues to change with increased nationalism, genocide, hatred of people who are 'different' and wars to settle territorial differences. All these make the need to hold onto one's identity and rituals even more important. It is the natural responsibility of parents/guardians and elders in society to make sure that these cultural norms are passed on from one generation to the next. This process of transmitting cultural norms to the next generation (enculturation) suggests that culture is something you are not born with but learn as you grow up. You learned your initial values and beliefs from your parents, the society you grew up in, the people you socialised and played with and went to school with. Enculturation is therefore important for the survival and continuation of generations and their identities. Living in a multicultural society, however, can interfere with this process.

Modification of culture

Natural transmission of culture from one generation to the next has often offered insurance that deeply held values and beliefs are carried forward in different communities and societies at large. For example, the stoicism of the Germans and 'stiff upper lip' found among the British continues despite exposure to different belief systems. The exposure to different cultural belief systems inevitably tends to modify the existing cultural norms found in enculturation, and it is true that the British 'upper lip' may not now be as 'stiff' as it was in Victorian times. Such modification is often referred to as acculturation, which suggests that different cultural groups may adapt their original views, values and beliefs following exposure to other cultures. Such exposure takes place in different ways and at different times. For example, education is often seen as the first and most fundamental modifier of parental-inspired values and belief systems (Nyatanga 2008a).

Education has the power to liberate minds and in some cases can lead to a revolution against parental influences, where these are viewed as restrictive or narrow. So why might people end up modifying their cultural values and beliefs? There are two key reasons for this. First, it is possible that people modify their cultural beliefs and behaviours in order to survive in their environment. For example, small groups of immigrants settling in the UK may have no choice but to modify in order to survive. They need to speak the language, communicate with health care professionals and engage with the etiquette of the host culture. Failure to do so might mean they remain at the periphery and are therefore marginalised in society.

Scenario

Imagine you attend university with a student from eastern Europe, who speaks good English but insists in talking to you in his mother tongue to help you to learn it. He even goes to the extent of contributing in lectures in his own language when explaining difficult concepts. He came to the UK before the referendum in June 2016 and now thinks everyone in the UK hates foreigners because he was sent abusive texts soon after the referendum results from unidentified senders telling him to 'go back home'. When you talk to him he implies that everyone (including you) is racist, but without actually saying it. He believes that his insistence on speaking in his own language might have created the hate texts and now does not trust anyone.

Here is an example of someone who does not want to engage with the English language publicly although he is fluent in it. His own beliefs are guiding his thinking, and may not outweigh the benefits and limitations of his behaviour. The outcome of the Brexit referendum seems to have made him 'paranoid' although it is certainly true that other people have received similar texts. What has happened here – and this is the real problem – is the generalisation that everyone, including you, does not want him around. We cannot understand an entire people through one person's experience or story. It is important to get more than one story/experience before we make generalisations. However, when you read newspaper reporting on racist attacks on foreign NHS staff increasing since June 2016, it is easy for foreigners to feel vulnerable even if this has not happened to them personally. For example, all broadsheet newspapers carried a story on 24 January 2017, stating that official figures show that there was more than one assult every day on non-white nurses, doctors and other frontline staff since the referendum. Yeung, reporting for *The Times* (2017), showed that assaults on NHS staff involving racial or religious factors rose by 271 in the year 2015–16, and by 320 by the end of October 2016. These reports suggest that both patients and staff with cultural, racial or religious differences may be vulnerable post-Brexit, and with that a negative impact of palliative care provision is possible. Staff of colour may care for patients with racist tendencies who are unpleasant to them and fail to appreciate their best care.

The second possible explanation may be that, once exposed to other cultures or life events, individuals may like or prefer some of the new values, such as equality for same sex marriage, and may modify their own beliefs accordingly. Acculturation is therefore a feature of multiculturalism and applies to both the minority and majority groups. It is important that we acknowledge that there are benefits and drawbacks to acculturation in a multicultural society.

Take some time now to think about what you already know about acculturation and make two separate lists:

- the benefits of acculturation when caring for patients receiving palliative care;
- what you see as negative aspects of acculturation when caring for patients receiving palliative care.

The benefits and negatives can be for the individual, group of individuals or society at large.

As this activity is based on your own observations, there is no outline answer at the end of this chapter.

While completing Activity 4.3 you may have found that acculturation not only brings benefits for patients but also challenges you as a health care professional. You could argue that acculturation brings about closer integration between different cultural groups. With integration comes a better understanding of each other's values and beliefs systems. When this happens, care delivered will most certainly meet the needs of the different patients we care for, and hopefully we can ensure dignity and a unique death. When acculturation happens in palliative care, it increases the need for cultural competence in the care we give to dying patients. When

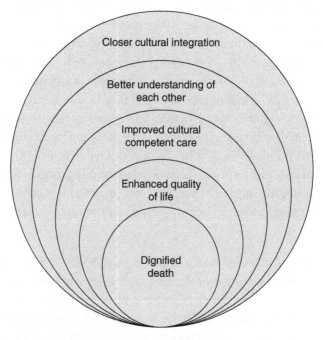

Figure 4.1: Benefits of acculturation.

completing Activity 4.3 you may have recognised that you need to develop your own cultural competence which you could find both exciting and alarming. Cultural competence will be discussed in more depth later in this chapter.

Figure 4.1 gives a summary of the benefits of acculturation. It emphasises that recognising acculturation and incorporating each aspect into the end of life care you offer your patients will increase the likelihood of your being able to ensure them a dignified death. It is important however to look at the bigger picture, as well as, most importantly, considering the impact of this on the patient. It is also clear from Table 4.2 that there are drawbacks of acculturation. Some are quite subtle, like loss of identity, while others are more apparent, such as overt peer pressure to behave or dress in a certain way. The point that needs making from this is that both benefits and drawbacks need closer integration if we are to achieve the best outcome (the best death) for dying patients.

Drawbacks
Threat to or loss of cultural identity
Modifying to survive and possible resentment
Challenges of multiple modifications
Much harder on older generations, therefore may 'cling' to traditional values

Table 4.2: Drawbacks of acculturation

Case study

Ahmed John-Paul, a 24-year-old single half Syrian, half Afghan man, migrates to the UK to escape war in Syria. He is a nurse by training but cannot work here. This is his first time in the UK and he speaks relatively good English, having spent two years working with an Australian in Aleppo. He has no relatives in the UK, and although the decision by the the UK government to bring him to the UK is on the whole beneficial for his career and life prospects, he has a few things to get used to. He needs to adjust quickly to the cold weather, since he arrived in January. The days are short and it gets dark around 5pm. He needs to get used to the different foods. Ahmed will need to 'pick up' the language very quickly in order to be able to communicate effectively with other people where he is living. Ahmed needs to understand the etiquette in order to socialise with others, make friends and maybe to find love. To achieve all this will take time, effort and resilience. Without the right support for Ahmed, this transition may be uncomfortable and he may often feel homesick.

While Ahmed is trying to settle into a new world here, there is disturbing news on the BBC that another young man who arrived in the UK at the same time as Ahmed has been arrested for possessing bomb-making material, has links to the terrorist group ISIS, and was preparing an attack on British soil.

The case study demonstrates that most people who migrate to another country have to make adjustments. For Ahmed, his migration was not his choosing and therefore he has no control over many things, like where to settle, which house, apartment, cottage to stay in and for how long. Adjustments help people like Ahmed to survive in the new environment and also to appreciate differences in so many areas, such as way of life, food and language. For Ahmed, anything is better than living under the threat of bombings and death in Aleppo. However, when people have no choice but to modify, this can threaten their own identity. Identity is what people try and protect when different groups of people meet, as it is that which distinguishes them from others. In this case Ahmed's identity may be endangered by the young man who has been arrested as he is associated to Ahmed through the group that came together to the UK. People watching or listening to the news may quickly and easily believe that all immigrants, and young men in particular, are abusing the kindness of the UK and now plan to perpetrate terrorist atrocities; and Ahmed by default falls into this group. If for some reason Ahmed needed health care intervention, he might find it difficult to feel free to access the services. However, more important is the question of how you, as the health care professional, would 'feel' treating Ahmed if he eventually accessed your service. It is important that you act in a professional way all the time, assess his needs and offer appropriate intervention.

Cultural competence in a world of multiculturalism

Everyone has an ethnic 'something' about them, and some people find themselves in the minority as a group when compared to other ethnic groups; therefore they are referred to as minority ethnic groups. Normally the colour of their skin and country of origin are used to differentiate their ethnic group (e.g., Black African, Black British or White Irish minority ethnic). This is neither a right nor an accurate way to describe people of different ethnic backgrounds. When you consider how the future generation coming out of a multicultural society might present, some of the terms used at present will be redundant and therefore meaningless. For example, with new family configurations, future generations of patients may defy traditional conceptions of culture and ethnicity, and therefore classifications used today may no longer be helpful in terms of what they tell us about difference among people.

This may mean a gradual blurring or loss of clear ethnic and cultural boundaries on which the current idea of cultural competence is based. The point is that, although cultural competence may remain a noble aspiration for health care professionals to achieve, this should be placed in the context of the changing cultural world of mass immigration, crosscultural fertilisation and marriages. It is from such changes that future assessments, service provision and palliative care may require different approaches to understand emerging cultural groups in order to continue to achieve cultural competence. However, the few changes highlighted above may in themselves add to the debate to invalidate the claim of achieving cultural competence for future generations. While it is helpful for you to understand traditional cultures, it is also crucial to recognise that even after considerable acculturation, most cultures will revert to their original values and

White British	White Irish	White other	White & Black Caribbean
White & Black African	White & Asian	Other mixed	Indian & Asian/ British Asian
Asian & British Asian/Pakistani	Asian & British Asian/ Bangladeshi	Other Asian	Black Caribbean & Black British
Black African & Black British	Other Black	Chinese	Any other group

Figure 4.2: Who are you?

beliefs when it comes to births, marriages and death rituals. These events are seen as significant in palliative care where you tend to witness death and dying rituals. Therefore it is crucially important that you also understand those original cultural values that existed before any acculturation took place.

One of the first and also most important things we do in order to understand the needs of our patients is to make an initial assessment on admission to our caseload. We collect a lot of data, including medical history and also ethnic and cultural background. This information is used for different purposes, including formulating the patient's plan of care. Figure 4.2 shows some of the options patients are asked to choose from, and you might have come across similar forms during your clinical placements.

Because of the complexity of accurately capturing patients' cultural backgrounds, there is a need to review how we assess patients' needs. Most writers, including Stiefel et al. (2017) and Nyatanga (2008a, 2011), now advocate focusing on the patient as a person and not as a cultural being. Rather than keeping on developing new tools for assessing patients from different cultural groups, it may work out better for both sides if student nurses and newly qualified staff are helped to feel confident enough to ask patients what matters most to them and how you can best help them.

For example, you could ask: What brings you here today? What is bothering you the most? Can you help me understand what is worrying you (if you think there could be psycho-social issues) or bothering you (if you suspect physical issues like pain) so that you can support them. It may also be proactive caring to ask direct questions to your patient. For example; Do you have any rituals/practices that I should be aware of in order to help you with your illness while you are with us?

What is important here is to think of what it is we are trying to understand by ascertaining ethnic/cultural background, and what we intend to do with the information. Apart from acquiring statistical information about the different types (cultural groups) of patients accessing and receiving care, other reasons are dubious. Even with the statistical need, we have to ask whether the information is accurately reflecting these patient groups. From the example in Figure 4.2, the information obtained could not be relied upon in terms of its accuracy. The next activity invites you to consider the importance of asking patients about their cultural background during nursing assessments.

Activity 4.4   *Critical thinking*

Look at the options presented to patients in Figure 4.2. What changes could you make so that this assessment yields the most accurate information for you as the nurse? Compare and note differences between this assessment form and the one used on the ward you are currently working (worked recently).

In general, the idea of understanding ethnic/cultural backgrounds helps to inform the information held by the Office for National Statistics, which is also responsible for the country's census, the latest being in 2011. In health care, assessing for ethnic/cultural breakdown helps us to understand disease patterns among different groups of the population. Different ethnic groups are prone to certain illnesses. For example, black African men over 50 years of age are more likely to develop prostate cancer (**www.prostatecanceruk.org**) when compared to other ethnic groups, and this is important in planning appropriate interventions.

For health care policy makers, commissioners and service providers, obtaining ethnic/cultural information helps to create a picture of which groups of the population access their services, and tailor the care to their cultural needs. It is clear that there are good intentions for assessing ethnic backgrounds of patients, but, as already discussed above, we have to be mindful that such information may, at some point, be inaccurate because of the cultural modifications through crosscultural fertilisation. This trend is not slowing down but increasing with increased migration, therefore the notion of cultural competence needs to be revised in line with the changing world picture.

Way forward

It is neither possible nor necessary to recommend a single solution that will meet every patient's need. Equality is not demonstrated by offering everyone a cup of coffee; rather, it can be achieved by offering everyone a drink of their choice. Cultural competence is no different in palliative care, as the needs of patients with the same cultural backgrounds may be different. The needs and wishes at death tend to expose the differences inherent in patients, and that is what is important for you to understand for your patient. In palliative care, what seems common is death and dying first, and then cultural influences. Therefore, if you start by talking openly about death and dying (Nyatanga 2013), you may find what is important to the patient first (some of which may be cultural) like practical issues, followed by controlling their pain. My natural inclination, and quite possibly yours as well, would be to address their pain first, but at times you may have to follow what the patient is asking you to do first. This is one example of putting aside our own values and beliefs and tailoring our help and support towards patients' wants and aspirations. Although this can be hard to do as a health care professional, it is true patient-centred care.

I have argued elsewhere that talking openly about death and dying is seen as one major step towards achieving a unique death, as desired by the dying patient (Nyatanga 2013). By focusing on the patient as a person and not a cultural being, we recognise and respect the uniqueness of all patients, and thereby understand their needs and aspirations for the remaining time of their life.

Recently, efforts to help people talk openly about death has resulted in the emergence of death cafés across the country and the Western world. The BBC Inside Out programme filmed parts of the activities of a death café as a way of raising awareness of death and helping to change attitudes (see the useful websites section at the end of the chapter).

The general understanding is that a death café gathering provides a platform to explore difficult questions and emotions surrounding our own death in an honest way in the company of non-judgemental others who are also seeking the same goals.

Activity 4.5 — *Reflection*

Using the link at the end of the chapter, watch the BBC coverage of death cafés and then reflect on your responses. Is a death café something you would use? Do you think a death café has benefits or drawbacks for the people who use them? Would you recommend a death café to your patients and their families? With each answer try and write down your reasons.

If the link at the end of the chapter fails to open, please read some ideas of a death café from the American site (also listed at the end of the chapter), and then attempt the activity.

Since this activity is based on your reflection there is no specific answer provided at the end. However, there is a brief discussion offered below.

Most people that I talk to about death cafés, including work colleagues, are bemused by the name itself. The bemusement comes from the combination of two very different concepts. Most people associate the word 'café' with food, drink and happiness, whereas death may not have these things in that order and meaning. People are drawn to death cafés for different reasons. For example, personal experiences of death, the effects of working with people experiencing death and dying or because they are uncomfortable thinking of death themselves. More fundamental reasons are about bringing social and cultural changes to society, about how death is viewed and to help normalise death as part of life. The bottom line is about changing views concerning death from being morbid to being a normal part of living. The outcome is about changing the way people deal with death (Prichep 2013) and bringing the topics of death and dying into an open conversation. However, before this can happen more evidence is needed to demonstrate that death cafés make a difference in people's approach to death and dying.

Looking deeper into the purpose of death cafés, inter alia, the following may signal a psychological leaning towards managing our own death anxiety. Therefore, as a way of reflection, the death café can be viewed as:

- a strategy that drives us to take away the grip death has over us (our conscious);
- a way to help us stop fearing death;
- a platform to normalise death as part of living;
- a way to free ourselves from the mental slavery of constantly denying death when it is a certainty for us all.

Finally, it is also important to consider the idea of 'meet me halfway', which requires both patients and health care professionals to make an effort to get to know each other. 'Meet me halfway' is a simple but effective concept that tries to educate people on values and beliefs that guide our different lives. To be successful, the concept requires closer integration by minority ethnic communities into wider society, learning the language and appreciating the social etiquette inherent in that society. Equally, the major culture (society) needs to be sensitive to the needs of minority groups. What tends to happen is that we can turn cultural differences into societal strength as we begin to work closely together.

It is therefore important that introspection takes place in an honest way so that we can understand ourselves in the face of difference. Consider the following message:

Why should I bother to get to know someone different? What is different means there is something new out there for us to explore. Something we can learn from, not with prejudice or fear but with respect and openness – so WHY NOT?
(Ann Fenech)

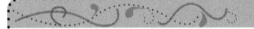

Chapter summary

This chapter has discussed a number of issues to do with culture and the need to care for every patient in a way that they prefer. Understanding patients' needs and preferences forms the basis of the understanding required to provide supportive palliative care. We discussed the term culture, which is often used loosely and therefore lacks a clear definition. For example, socially, culture may refer to music trends, dance types, food and drink, clothes, sex, sports and other hobbies. In health care, culture may refer to a way of caring in a particular hospital or ward/unit or out in the community. As a society, we may use the term culture to refer to race, nationality, ethnicity, rituals, heritage and traditions. It is clear from the above that culture refers to different things about people's characteristics – behaviour, preferences or rituals. The culture we are most concerned with in the context of this book is that which guides how different patients and family pursue their values and belief systems, leading to how they prefer to be cared for and die. The important point we discussed was that understanding one patient in this way helps us to understand that every patient is unique, therefore they will all have different concerns as they approach death.

We discussed the impact of acculturation on individual patients and also on us as health care professionals. This led us into the idea of multicultural society and how health care professionals can be competent when caring in such an environment. This led to the discussion about the need for cultural competence and the challenges inherent in this idea. While cultural competence is a noble idea, the cultural world around it is changing and therefore we need to start planning for care that reflects the future. We concluded that we needed to achieve cultural competence in a different way; by focusing on the patient before us and understanding them as a person first and as a cultural being second. It is important that we learn from the experiences of palliative care providers already working closely with different cultural communities.

The idea of a death café is worth considering with an open mind, and maybe we need to experience one for ourselves before recommending them to others.

Finally, the increases in migration across Europe and the world at large is an important indicator that the world is changing. With that comes both positive outcomes (learning from each other, pooling of different skills, knowledge and values) and the negative re-emergence of nationalism, hatred and intolerance of difference which poses a huge challenge on you as the professional health care provider. As with many codes of conduct in health care, we all need to act in a professional way that does not discriminate, disadvantage or create bias towards another human being. Cultural difference should be viewed and taken as something new for us to explore openly and learn from.

Activities: brief outline answers

Activity 4.4: Critical thinking

- It is not clear what the different categories are trying to achieve, as these options are not the same (uniform). Some options, like white or black, focus on skin colour, whereas options like white and Asian refer to children of marriages between these two groups. The other options focus on country of birth/origin, like: Pakistani, Indian, British and Bangladeshi, while others refer to continents where people come from, like Asian, African. It is important to point out that the patient may have had his/her values influenced by different backgrounds, and therefore the range of options in this activity may not accurately capture all of the patient's cultural background. Consequently, the care offered and services provided may be based on inaccurate information. This may explain why most people from the BME community still do not access the palliative care services that are on offer in the UK. They perceive services as unacceptable and not addressing their needs.
- One final point to make is the 'Other' option, as it is hard to make sense of who this group is and their values. This othering label suggests they are not important enough to be allocated their own group.

Further reading

Gilbert, P. (ed.) (2013) *Spirituality and End of Life Care.* Hove: Pavillion Publishing.

Although the title is spirituality, this book discusses important aspects of end of life care. For example, there are chapters on a good death as well as on dignity in end of life care. You may find Parts 1–5 most relevant as you start your new career in nursing and palliative care.

Oliviere, D., Munroe, B. and Payne, S. (2011) *Death, Dying, and Social Differences*, 2nd edn. Oxford: Oxford University Press.

This book discusses key aspects of cultural, ethnic and social differences. It is relevant to palliative care, and is written by experts in the field. It is easy to read and informative.

Yeung, P. (2017) Racist assaults on hospital staff double in a year. *The Times*, 24 January 2017. Available from: www.thetimes.co.uk/article/brexit-blamed-for-soaring-assaults-on-hospital-staff-tbpwxg397 (accessed 30 March 2017).

Useful websites

www.ons.gov.uk/census

This website provides a gateway to national statistics of the UK's population. It gives an overview of the UK population, its size, characteristics and the causes of population change including national and regional variation and including net immigration, gender differences and life expectancy.

http://prostatecanceruk.org/

This website is owned by Prostate Cancer UK, and aims to raise awareness about prostate cancer. It encourages men (black in particular), with the support of their families, to be tested early for the disease. It also gives information on developments and recommended treatments.

http://deathcafe.com/what/

The site introduces the concept of a death café and shows a 6 minute video clip of someone describing how they started to encourage others to talk about death openly.

www.bbc.co.uk/iplayer/episode/b07tc0bw/inside-out-west-midlands-12092016

The BBC Inside Out programme on death cafés.

www.agingcare.com/articles/death-cafe-grab-a-drink-talk-about-death-159860.htm

Information on death cafés in America.

Chapter 5
Rehabilitation in palliative and end of life care

Jane Nicol

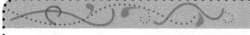

NMC Standards for Pre-registration Nursing Education

This chapter will address the following competencies:

Domain 1: Professional values

4. All nurses must work in partnership with service users, carers, families, groups, communities and organisations. They must manage risk, and promote health and wellbeing while aiming to empower choices that promote self care and safety.

6. All nurses must understand the roles and responsibilities of other health and social care professionals, and seek to work with them collaboratively for the benefit of all who need care.

Domain 4: Leadership, management and team working

7. All nurses must work effectively across professional and agency boundaries, actively involving and respecting others' contributions to integrated person-centred care. They must know when and how to communicate with and refer to other professionals and agencies in order to respect the choices of service users and others, promoting shared decision-making, to deliver positive outcomes and to coordinate smooth, effective transition within and between services and agencies.

NMC Essential Skills Clusters

This chapter will address the following ESCs:

Cluster: Organisational aspects of care

9. People can trust the newly registered graduate nurse to treat them as partners and work with them to make a holistic and systematic assessment of their needs; to develop a personalised plan that is based on mutual understanding and respect for their individual situation promoting health and wellbeing, minimising risk of harm and promoting their safety at all times.

By the second progression point

10. With the person and under supervision, plans safe and effective care by recording and sharing information based on the assessment.

continued ... •

By entry to the register

15. Works within the context of a multiprofessional team and works collaboratively with other agencies when needed to enhance the care of people, communities and populations.

16. Promotes health and wellbeing, self care and independence by teaching and empowering people and carers to make choices in coping with the effects of treatment and the ongoing nature and likely consequences of a condition including death and dying.

10. People can trust the newly registered graduate nurse to deliver nursing interventions and evaluate their effectiveness against the agreed assessment and care plan.

By the second progression point

1. Acts collaboratively with people and their carers enabling and empowering them to take a shared and active role in the delivery and evaluation of nursing interventions.

By entry to the register

6. Provides safe and effective care in partnership with people and their carers within the context of people's ages, conditions and developmental stages.

14. People can trust the newly registered graduate nurse to be an autonomous and confident member of the multi-disciplinary or multi agency team and to inspire confidence in others.

By the second progression point

3. Values others' roles and responsibilities within the team and interacts appropriately.

By entry to the register

6. Actively consults and explores solutions and ideas with others to enhance care.

10. Works inter-professionally and autonomously as a means of achieving optimum outcomes for people.

Chapter aims

After reading this chapter you will be able to:

- apply the domains of holistic care to your practice;
- recognise the role rehabilitation has in palliative and end of life care;
- use goal setting to promote rehabilitation, and improve quality of life, for people receiving palliative and end of life care;
- understand the concept of 'survivorship' and the role rehabilitation has in this.

Introduction

There are still so many things I'd like to do, not big things, just everyday things, meet with friends, cook a meal – things that until I had COPD (chronic obstructive pulmonary disease) I took for granted. Now, I can't always see how I can carry on doing these.

Years ago a diagnosis of cancer was nearly always fatal, that's not the case now. I was diagnosed with bowel cancer 6 years ago, had surgery and chemotherapy … now I have a yearly check up and I've been told that will stop soon. That worries me a bit.

These quotes illustrate the changing face of health care, both in the UK and globally. Improved medical treatment and ongoing care now mean that people, who would previously have lived with more debilitating symptoms or would have died, are living longer. In the first quote you can see that the person has a desire to maintain their independence, to be able to continue to do the things that provide their life with meaning and to contribute to shared experiences. In the second quote the person whose treatment was successful has concerns about their future. This may seem strange to you; you may feel that having survived their diagnosis and treatment they should be celebrating their recovery. However, after years of ongoing treatment, living with the consequences of this and with the support given to them, for some the realisation that this will stop may be seen as a personal loss and trigger feelings of bereavement (see Chapter 3 for further information on loss, grief and bereavement).

These quotes recognise two very different situations. In the first the person is likely to die as a result of their long term condition while the second person is more likely to 'survive' their condition. However, one thing is certain: they will both require support to enable them to 'live well'. Research has shown that many of the priorities people receiving palliative care have focus on 'living', with being able to 'take charge' seen as an overarching theme (Carter et al. 2003). One aspect of this is related to symptom management and life functioning with participants recognising the need for balance between when to 'pace' and 'push' themselves. Rehabilitation, whether physical, social, emotional or psychological, can be seen as a means by which to support people to 'take charge'.

For rehabilitation to be effective it is important for you to recognise that a person is not just a body, but is a 'whole' person with a mind, body and spirit that are interconnected in a way that affects the person's sense of wellbeing and 'hope'. This holistic approach to care requires you to be self-aware and to work with people, their carers and families to promote the delivery of care that addresses the needs of the 'whole' person.

Defining holistic care

Holistic nursing care embraces the mind, body and spirit of the patient, in a culture that supports a therapeutic nurse/patient relationship, resulting in wholeness, harmony and healing. Holistic care is patient led and patient focused in order to provide individualised care, thereby, caring for the patient as a whole person rather than in fragmented parts.
(McEvoy and Duffy 2008: 418)

The term 'holism' comes from the Greek work *holos*, which means whole. Holistic care has been part of nursing practice for decades and can find its roots in humanist theories where patients were viewed as unique individuals continually interacting with their environment (Rogers 1970; Levine 1971). Today this means viewing the patient as a whole, recognising the interconnection between the physical, social, cultural and spiritual aspects and the impact that illness can have on these (McEvoy and Duffy 2008). In their concept analysis of holistic nursing practice, McEvoy and Duffy (2008) identified the following recurring characteristics of holism:

- mind – the emotional and social aspect of a person;
- body – the physical aspect of a person;
- spirit – the spiritual and cultural aspect of a person;
- whole – recognising the person as a whole and the interrelation between mind, body and spirit;
- harmony – working in partnership with the patient;
- healing – recognising what is important to the patient and addressing these aspects.

The following case study illustrates how these characteristics relate to holistic care.

Case study

Gurpreet is a 45-year-old man who has high grade non-Hodgkin's lymphoma. He has been receiving chemotherapy treatment for this and was recently admitted to hospital with pyrexia and a consistently low white cell count. Here is a narrative from one of the nurses looking after Gurpreet.

When I met Gurpreet for the first time, the first thing he said to me was 'when can I go home?' [mind and healing]. *He went on to explain that it was his youngest son's birthday in 2 days' time and that he really wanted to be home by then to celebrate with family and friends* [mind and spirit]. *My initial reaction was to reassure Gurpreet* [healing] *without raising his hopes* [whole]. *I told him that, though he may not be home in time for his son's birthday, he would be discharged as soon as he was stable* [healing and whole]. *I then asked Gurpreet if I could take a set of observations to see how his temperature and other vital signs were* [body and harmony].

As I started to take Gurpreet's pulse he began to talk to me, asking about his pyrexia and white cell count and whether this would mean his chemotherapy would have to stop. I immediately stopped what I was doing [whole, healing and harmony]. *I sat down and let Gurpreet continue to talk; he was especially worried about how to talk to his children about his current health* [mind and spirit] *and the fact that he might miss his son's birthday party had brought the reality of his situation home to him* [whole].

I asked Gurpreet if his family were receiving any support [mind and harmony] *and whether this was something that he would like to consider* [healing]. *I told him about the family and children support groups at the local hospice, reassuring him that it is not just for the families of people who are dying, but for any family where someone has a potentially life limiting condition* [whole, harmony and healing]. *Gurpreet's face visibly relaxed at this point* [mind and spirit] *and he asked for more information, which I said I was happy to provide* [harmony and healing] *and said I would return with more information* [healing].

The above case study demonstrates how seemingly small interactions can have a profound impact on the person and their sense of wellbeing. It is clear from the case study that the nurse recognised that Gurpreet wanted to talk and then allowed him to lead the conversation and gauge how much information he was given. You should remember that not everyone will wish to discuss their social, cultural and spiritual lives. They may feel it is not necessary to their care; indeed, they may feel it is intrusive. It is important therefore that you know the people you are nursing, how much they are prepared to share with you and whether what you are asking them impacts on the care you deliver.

Activity 5.1   *Reflection*

Using a reflection from your clinical practice that was based on a patient interaction, integrate the characteristics of holism (mind, body, spirit, whole, harmony and healing) to your reflection.

Brief answers to all activities are given at the end of the chapter, unless otherwise indicated. This activity is based on your own observations, so there is no outline answer given.

You can see from the case study and Activity 5.1 that the relationship between the technical care provided and how this care is carried out is central to holistic care. Once you recognise the importance of both these aspects your care will include both the science and art of nursing, especially important for providing person-centred rehabilitation in palliative and end of life care.

Changing demographics and disease trajectories at end of life

Due to changing demographics and disease incidence, health care services including the National Health Service, tertiary and charitable organisations have to respond proactively. The population of the UK is getting older; the number of people over the age of 85 is expected to double by 2025 to 3.5 million (ONS 2011). This ageing population means that it is more likely that people will be living with one or more long term conditions, requiring complex ongoing care and management; it is expected that the number of people living with one or more long term conditions will rise to 2.9 million in 2018 (DH 2012).

This is reflected in the changing scope of palliative and end of life care as it extends beyond cancer care and support with services supporting an increasing number of people with long term conditions such as COPD, neurological conditions and cardiovascular disease. Indeed a report written by Calanzani et al. (2013) for Help the Hospices identified that by 2035 people aged over 85 will account for almost half of all deaths in the UK. This older population, with health needs that increase over time as their long term conditions deteriorate, face a slower progression towards death. These differing disease trajectories can make planning for palliative and end of life care challenging, though they do offer opportunities for rehabilitation.

To support you to care for people receiving palliative and end of life care it would be helpful for you to have an understanding of disease trajectories and how they differ. In 2002 Lunney et al. examined disease trajectories at end of life to determine if a person's functional decline differed depending on their type of illness. The four causes of death included were: sudden death, death from cancer, death from organ failure and frailty and cognitive decline. The results of their study concluded that functional decline varied at end of life depending on the illness; see Figure 5.1. As you can see from this their results showed that one of the most unpredictable trajectories was for organ failure. The disease trajectory in these cases is identified by episodes of exacerbation followed by periods of stabilisation with some functional decline in health.

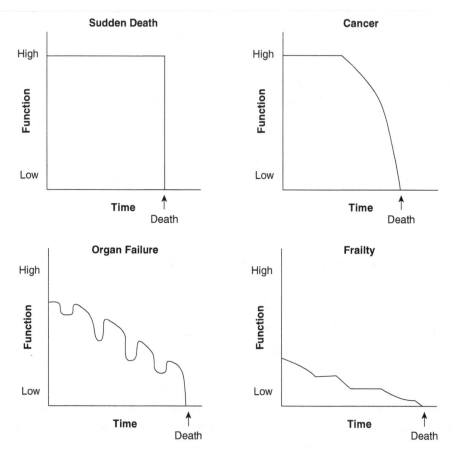

Figure 5.1: Trajectories of dying (Lunney et al. 2002).

Activity 5.2 — *Critical thinking*

Review the different disease trajectories outlined in Figure 5.1 and identify when rehabilitation could form part of a person's care and treatment.

As you can see from Activity 5.2 there is the potential for rehabilitation to form part of the ongoing care and management of people receiving palliative and end of life care. People may move between times when their care has a more palliative focus to a time when there is a more rehabilitative focus and vice versa.

Rehabilitation in palliative and end of life care

WHO (2012b) defines rehabilitation as:

> *a process aimed at enabling people with disabilities to reach and maintain their optimum physical, sensory, intellectual, psychological and social functional levels.*

Now consider the definition of palliative care given in Chapter 1 where there is an emphasis on improving the quality of life for people and their families. Given the central idea of both definitions you can begin to identify a clear interface between the two. This is further echoed in Dame Cicely Saunders' view of hospice care that emphasised a person achieving their 'maximum potential' through maintaining 'control and independence wherever possible' (Saunders 1998).

Recognising the changes discussed earlier in this chapter, in 2013 the Hospice UK Commission into the Future of Hospice Care asked hospices to consider how they will meet this challenge and to think critically about how they can meet the needs of this changing population. The report *Rehabilitative Palliative Care, Enabling People to Live Fully Until They Die, a Challenge for the 21st Century* (Tiberini and Richardson 2015) formed part of this commission. In this report rehabilitation, in the context of palliative and end of life care, is defined as:

> *a paradigm which integrates rehabilitation, enablement, self-management and self-care into the holistic model of palliative care.*

This focus on empowerment clearly places the person at the centre of the process. However, you should recognise that to achieve this there will need to be effective multidisciplinary support available that works collaboratively with the person and their family enabling them to adjust to ongoing losses and fulfil personal aspirations. Recognising the ongoing losses (see Chapter 3 for further exploration of loss, grief and bereavement) will encourage you to alter the focus of your rehabilitation as the person's condition deteriorates and their needs and aspirations change.

Phases of rehabilitation in palliative and end of life care

Having an understanding of the different phases of rehabilitation used in palliative and end of life care will support you to ensure that you provide personalised rehabilitation that focuses on the individual needs of the person. One of the first people to identify different phases of rehabilitation in palliative and end of life care was J. Herbert Deitz (1981). These are illustrated in Table 5.1.

While Deitz originally focused on oncology patients, you can see from Table 5.1 that in addition to cancer his phases of rehabilitation can be applied to a range of long term conditions. In Table 5.1 the focus of the rehabilitation goals has been in improving and maintaining the person's physical ability. This should not be addressed in isolation and you should always be mindful of addressing the emotional and psychological needs of the person. For example, while you might view the introduction of adaptive equipment and/or a wheelchair as a positive, this is not always

Phases of rehabilitation		
	Example of a goal to support the rehabilitation of a person living with motor neurone disease	
	Situation	**Goal**
Preventative: interventions that will reduce the effect of expected disabilities	Due to their diagnosis the person is at risk of muscle fatigue and wasting	To actively participate in pre-diagnosis exercise activity or to start moderate exercise (both strengthening and aerobic) – ongoing
Restorative: interventions that aim to return the person to their previous level of function	There is potential for the person to regain strength to walk short distances, maximum of 5 metres and to manage 2 steps	To regain the ability to stand and walk safely, on a level surface (consider the use of adaptive equipment, e.g., leg brace) – 2 weeks
Supportive: interventions that teach people how to accommodate their disability and focus on maximising function and independence	Due to further loss of muscle strength and coordination the person is no longer able to walk	To promote independence through maintaining the person's ability to stand and transfer from bed to chair independently (consider the use of adaptive equipment, e.g., swivel cushions, wheelchair) – both short term (2 weeks) and ongoing
Palliative: interventions aimed at minimising complications, providing comfort and supporting adjustment to a new reality	The person is no longer able to transfer and will not regain this function	To reduce complications of reduced mobility through teaching pressure-relieving techniques to the person and their family and correct limb splinting – ongoing

Table 5.1: Deitz (1981) phases of rehabilitation and their application to clinical practice

the case for the person. They may see this introduction as a reminder of what they have lost and are still to lose. Therefore, how you present this to the person is important. Introducing a wheelchair as a way of promoting independence and maintaining safety can help reduce the negative impact.

Activity 5.3   *Critical thinking*

Using the information in Table 5.1 read the following case study. Throughout this case study you are asked to consider what the focus and aim of your rehabilitation would be. In all tasks think about which aspects of holistic care you are addressing.

Chris is 51 years old, single and lives alone. As a long distance lorry driver, he works long hours and is often away from home for periods of time. His next of kin is his sister who lives 300 miles away.

Five years ago during a routine health check Chris was diagnosed with hypertension and high choles-terol. He takes an ace inhibitor (enalapril) and cholesterol lowering medication (simvastatin) daily. Chris does not exercise regularly and over the past few years has put on weight. In addition to a lack of exercise Chris smokes; he has tried to stop in the past but has not been successful.

Two days ago he had an episode of chest pain and was admitted to hospital where he was prescribed and commenced on aspirin, a beta blocker and GTN for when he has chest pain. This episode scared Chris and he is feeling vulnerable and frustrated by his situation.

Task one

Preventative rehabilitation: you are working on the ward where Chris is receiving treat-ment and are planning his care; what would the focus and aim of your rehabilitation be?

Chris is now 63 years old. In addition to living with cardiovascular disease 18 months ago he was diagnosed with COPD. He continues to smoke, though has managed to lose some weight, though his BMI is still high. Chris has just been discharged from hospital following treatment for pneumonia; he was in hospital for three weeks, is feeling weak and has lost muscle tone in his legs making it difficult for him to walk. He is attending an appointment with the community physiotherapist with whom you are spending the day.

Task two

Restorative rehabilitation: given Chris's current situation what would the aim of your reha-bilitation be at this point? What members of the health care team might you involve in this?

Chris's condition is deteriorating; he is now 68 years old and has been admitted to hospital three times in the past eight months due to episodes of chest pain that his GTN spray did not resolve. His medica-tion has been reviewed and he has been prescribed a calcium channel blocker and a diuretic as he now has some signs of cardiac failure. He remains overweight and finds it difficult to mobilise due to pain in his legs and breathlessness.

continued …

Task three

Supportive rehabilitation: you are on a primary care placement with Chris's district nurse team and are visiting Chris. As Chris's symptoms worsen and his level of ability reduces, what would be the aim of rehabilitation at this point? What adaptive equipment might you introduce?

Chris is being cared for at home by the primary health care team. Over the past 18 months his condition has continued to deteriorate. He is no longer able to mobilise and has carers coming in twice a day. He has expressed a preference to stay at home. His pain is stable, though he finds his breathlessness quite distressing. He has been prescribed 500mcgs lorazepam for this.

Task four

Palliative rehabilitation: you are visiting Chris with his palliative care nurse specialist; what is the focus of your rehabilitation?

Completing Activity 5.3 will have encouraged you to identify the role rehabilitation has throughout a person's disease trajectory. Up to this point we have looked at the broad concept of rehabilitation and its role in palliative and end of life care and have identified how you can use this in your clinical practice. To encourage you to address rehabilitation more specifically the next section of this chapter will look at goal setting as a means to support you to provide rehabilitation that clearly meets the needs of people receiving palliative and end of life care.

Goal setting in rehabilitation

Goal setting or goal planning is seen as a cornerstone of effective rehabilitation and has been for many years. In the 1960s Edwin Locke was the first to put forward a specific goal setting theory. His theory proposed that setting goals is motivational and that people will work harder when the goal is more challenging (Locke and Latham 2002). However, for this to be achievable, when setting goals it is important that you take into consideration the person's belief about whether they can achieve the goal or not; this is known as their self-efficacy (Locke and Latham 2002). This means the person has to view any goals that are set as ones they can realistically achieve, resulting in high self-efficacy and motivation. Conversely, if unrealistic goals are set and the person can see they are not achieving them, their self-efficacy and motivation reduces making it even less likely they will achieve their goal, and be willing to participate in goal setting in the future.

While goal setting is well established as a part of 'traditional' rehabilitation, there is a lack of consensus in the research about the appropriateness of its use in palliative care.

Research summary: goal setting in palliative care

In 2014 Boa et al. published their structured review of goal setting in palliative care. They searched multiple electronic databases for papers that focused on: *patient centred goal setting for patients with advanced, progressive life threatening illness.* They did not limit their search to a specific type of paper, date of publication or research methodology. Boa et al. recognised the challenges of being able to systematically review such diverse data. To address this they used Hawker et al.'s (2002) review method which was specifically designed for the systematic appraisal of diverse data.

To ensure that papers met the required inclusion/exclusion criteria all suitable papers were read in full by at least two of the authors. Critical appraisal of the papers using Hawker et al.'s (2002) tool was carried out, independently, by two authors; where agreement could not be reached a third reviewer arbitrated. This process ensured that all papers were judged fairly and reduced the likelihood of reviewer influence and associated bias. Each paper was read closely; recurrent and relevant topics were identified and, through discussion with all authors, reviewed until agreement was reached. Sixteen papers were included in the review, with three themes being identified:

Definitions, process and functions of goal setting – their findings confirmed goals should be personalised and involve partnership working between the person, their family/carer and the health care professionals. In addition many of the papers identified that people review their goals as their condition deteriorates. Health care professionals may see some person identified goals as unrealistic, however this approach may support people to realise what is and what is not achievable and adjust accordingly, providing the person with a sense of control over their situation. Findings also proposed that for some people the process of setting goals was just as important as achieving them.

The challenges of delivering goal setting in palliative care – this theme highlighted the difficulty in using goal setting in palliative and end of life care without adjustment. In part this is due to the fact that in 'traditional' rehabilitation the likelihood is the person will return to their previous level of function, whereas in palliative care the person is faced with a gradual decline in function which is often unpredictable. This indicates that goal setting in palliative care should be responsive to the person's deteriorating condition with goals redefined if required. It was also identified that the focus of the person's goals change as their condition deteriorates with goals moving from improving physical function to goals about leaving a personal legacy. Interestingly in this theme it was identified that some health care professionals find it difficult to support people who have set 'unrealistic goals'. Given the potential importance of this for a person, as identified in the first theme, any negotiation of goals must be collaborative and empower the person.

Theories underpinning goal setting – hope was a concept that reoccurred in the articles included in the review, with hope being what a person believes their future possibilities are.

(Continued)

(Continued)

To maintain a person's hopefulness setting specific goals is important as this allows ongoing monitoring of the goal and achievement. What is important is finding the balance between 'hope', what a person could achieve, and 'expectation', what a person will achieve; acknowledging this interplay could support health care professionals to find a compromise. Here non-achievement of a goal is seen as an opportunity to increase a person's resilience through the development of new goals.

The authors recognise the limitations of their review; this was the first time a structured review of goal setting in palliative care was undertaken. In addition while the authors made every attempt to ensure a rigorous appraisal process, thematic analysis is a subjective process and they acknowledge other researchers may have identified different themes.

Throughout this chapter it has been acknowledged that rehabilitation in palliative and end of life care is an area that needs to be developed further. The research presented in this summary goes towards providing an evidence base on which to develop rehabilitation in palliative care as an integral part of palliative and end of life care. The research summary above identifies the importance of setting specific goals, ensuring these are, where possible, achievable and including ongoing review of any goals set. An approach that will support you to do this is to set SMART goals.

Setting SMART goals

Setting SMART goals means that you are assisting the person to set goals that are: Specific, Measurable, Achievable, Realistic and Timed. Using this acronym can help guide the detail of the goal to be achieved (see Table 5.2).

	SMART goals
Specific	Clearly defines what the goal is: instead of saying 'I'm going to eat less' say 'On weekdays I'm not going to eat snacks after my evening meal'.
Measurable	Identifies what progress towards the goal is and if it has been achieved: 'eat less' is not measurable, but 'on weekdays I'm not going to eat snacks after my evening meal' is, both in terms of time spend and achievement.
Achievable	Explore this from the person's point of view and your own; ask them to rate how much they believe they can achieve their goal. Rating their belief out of 10 will provide you with an indicator as to whether they believe the goal is achievable. For successful achievement you would be looking for the person to rate their belief as 7 or above.

Realistic	Being realistic about the goal and the timeframe for the goal will ensure that the goal is achievable.
Timed	Setting a date for achievement provides a focus; it also encourages the person to consider if the goal is realistic and achievable, which may result in the goal being reviewed. Timeframes should be considered in relation to the person's usual day-to-day activities.

Table 5.2: SMART goals

In addition to the information in Table 5.2 it is important that you find out the person's current level of ability, e.g., how far can the person currently walk, on what type of ground (flat, slope), can they manage stairs, are they able to wash and dress themselves, are they independent in some aspects of this, e.g., brushing teeth, dressing their top half? You can then use this as a benchmark against which the person can review their progress and achievement.

Activity 5.4   *Decision-making*

Esther is 60 years old. She lives with her husband and son in a two-bedroomed semi-detached house in a city suburb. Her husband is working as an engineer for the local council and her son works as a PE teacher at a local high school. Esther is currently living with the following long term conditions:

- *type 2 diabetes*
- *diabetic peripheral neuropathy*
- *cardiovascular disease.*

Esther was diagnosed with type 2 diabetes at the age of 42; at this time she was prescribed metformin and advised to reduce the amount of fat and sugar in her diet. Initially she managed to do this, however following the death of her other son at the age of 15, Esther became depressed; she did not leave the house and spent her time watching television and snacking. It was at this time she stopped work; she had been a receptionist at a local GP surgery. During this period her blood glucose level was regularly above 12 mmol/L. Gradually Esther's mental health improved and 18 months after her son's death she began to help out at the local gospel church lunch club.

Unfortunately at the age of 53 Esther was diagnosed with diabetic peripheral neuropathy, which affects the sensation in her hands and feet. This resulted in Esther having a non-healing ulcer on her left ankle, which required ongoing treatment over a long period. As part of her treatment she had negative pressure wound therapy; this improved her ulcer and since then it has not broken down again. Her neuropathy also affected her balance and her confidence in going outside. This meant that Esther reduced the amount of exercise she was taking, though she still helped out at the church lunch club as this was something that she enjoyed. She views this lunch club as her 'lifeline' as it provided her with a way to adjust to the death of her son.

continued ...

Four years ago Esther had a stroke, which left her with a right-sided weakness of both her arm and leg, and at this time she was started on medication to lower her cholesterol, aspirin and a beta blocker. Esther worked hard to regain her mobility following her stroke and until another stroke 3 weeks ago was able to attend to her activities of daily living, cooking the occasional meal for her family and helping out at the church lunch club. This second stroke has further weakened her right side (she currently needs the support of two people to transfer) and her speech has been affected (dysarthria). Esther is currently in the local community hospital.

You are working on the ward and have been caring for Esther during her stay and are working with Esther to increase her independence. You and Esther have identified the following areas as being part of Esther's rehabilitation:

- Increasing Esther's mobility – initially being able to transfer from her bed to chair independently (Esther scores her belief in being able to achieve this at 7).

Identify which phase of rehabilitation Esther is in, and compile a SMART goal that will allow Esther to achieve her aims and include relevant members of the health care team.

- Being able to return to helping at the church lunch club she is involved in.

Consider how this goal is to be achieved, if it is possible to compile a SMART goal for this or whether several shorter term goals will be required to enable Esther to achieve this goal. What members of the health care team might be involved in this goal? Consider which aspects of holism you are addressing in relation to this goal.

As you can see from Activity 5.4 people will have a range of short and long term goals that they would like to achieve. Setting shorter term goals provides focus for the person and means that they can see progress quickly; longer term goals provide something for the person to aim for. Very often longer term goals are the ones that add 'meaning' or 'quality' to the person's life. By providing ongoing feedback to the person about their progress towards their short term goals you will increase their sense of self belief and hope that they can succeed. As part of this you could also encourage the person to document their progress themselves, giving the person a sense of ownership over their goals and providing evidence of whether they are making progress or if they are needing some more assistance (Furze 2015). It is likely however that due to the nature of the person's condition this will continue to deteriorate and all goals may not be achievable. Despite this it is still important that you emphasise the positive aspects of what the person has achieved, even if goals are reviewed.

So far in this chapter the emphasis has been on the role of rehabilitation for patients receiving palliative and end of life care. However, as mentioned at the start of this chapter there are increasing numbers of people 'surviving' cancer. While not strictly palliative and end of life care the last part of this chapter will address 'survivorship' and the role of rehabilitation.

Survivorship: living with and beyond cancer

Isaac had undergone multiple surgeries, a post-operative wound infection, chemotherapy and radiation treatment. He was now a cancer survivor.

The term survivor indicates that some 'battle' has taken place and someone has won. Words synonymous with war are often used in relation to cancer: 'cancer fighting foods', 'he bravely fought cancer' and 'let's beat cancer sooner'. Terms like these are used by organisations working in the field of cancer research and support; the last one is the tag line on Cancer Research UK's 'support us' webpage. While terms like these can be a rallying call, for the person living with cancer, their families and friends and the general public, they do not always recognise the human cost to the person who has lived through this 'battle' and is still living. If you want to find out more about the term 'cancer survivor' and its perception among people who have 'survived cancer', read the article by Khan et al. (2012) listed in the further reading section at the end of this chapter.

Given the different views on the term 'survivor', many health care professionals prefer to use the term 'living with and beyond cancer' as it recognises that there is the potential for the person who has 'survived' to 'live well' with the ongoing impact of their diagnosis and recovery. This is the term that will be used here. Currently in the UK more than 2 million people are living with or beyond cancer, and this number is increasing by approximately 3 per cent every year. If this rate continues it is estimated 4 million people in the UK could be living with and beyond cancer by 2030 (Maddams et al. 2012). While this can be viewed positively, demonstrating the impact of improved research, screening and treatment, there is a very personal cost to this. How does a person who has been told they are 'cured' go and live their life; what is the impact of surviving cancer on that person? A Macmillan report published in 2013 estimated that as many as 500,000 people living with or beyond cancer live with one or more physical or psychological consequences of their cancer, or its treatment (Macmillan Cancer Support 2013).

Activity 5.5   *Critical thinking*

Take the time to consider the types of treatment people with cancer may have had and list some of the possible long term consequences, physical, social and emotional, of this.

By reviewing the consequences you listed in Activity 5.5 you can begin to identify the role rehabilitation has in supporting people to live with and beyond cancer to adapt to their new life. Macmillan Cancer Support (2014) has developed a competency framework aimed at enhancing nurses' confidence to provide support for people living with and beyond cancer (Table 5.3).

As you can see from Table 5.3 many of the competencies reflect the themes already identified in this chapter: holistic care, rehabilitation that is aimed at maintaining and improving

Domain	Application to practice
1. Clinical nursing practice	Nurses are required to have knowledge of cancer and its treatment, interpreting tests and investigations and participating in ongoing monitoring. Nurses must be able to carry out a holistic assessment of the person paying particular attention to medication management and symptom management
2. Care coordination	Nurses must be able to compile personalised care plans liaising with members of the health care team. This should include plans for transitional care, e.g., when a person is discharged from secondary to primary care
3. Proactive management	Nurses should support people to make informed choices; they should know the types of support and resources available and use this information to promote the participation of people in their own care acknowledging and respecting the decisions they make
4. Psychosocial wellbeing	Nurses are required to demonstrate understanding of the psychological effects of cancer and to use this information to support people to develop coping strategies, use strategies to assess psychological needs, e.g., concerns checklist and refer on to specialist services if needed
5. Identifying high-risk individuals	Nurses should be able to identify high-risk individuals and have an understanding of the factors that may increase a person's need for services, e.g., co-morbidities. Working collaboratively the nurse will help the person to identify strengths and weaknesses and how to address these to improve health and wellbeing
6. Supporting self-care, self-management and enabling independence	Nurses will promote self-management, through addressing lifestyle and behaviour choices, working in partnership, to put together a plan of care, using motivational interviewing and their knowledge of services to enable the person to make positive changes
7. Professional practice and leadership	Nurses should have the skills to participate in auditing services, understanding evidence-based practice and the research methodologies used and how these can impact on care and service development
8. Interagency and partnership working	Nurses are required to liaise with health care professionals and other agencies collaboratively; this includes statutory, non-statutory and voluntary organisations, e.g., housing, financial, vocational

Table 5.3: Macmillan Cancer Support competency framework for nurses (2014)

both functional ability and psychological adjustment, and goal setting. Whether providing rehabilitation for a person who will die or for a person who will 'survive', what is important is that you address their needs holistically and work in partnership with them and other health care professionals to provide rehabilitation that enables them to live well.

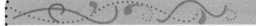

Chapter summary

This chapter has provided you with an overview of rehabilitation in palliative and end of life care. To promote person-centred care the term holistic care has been explored and the need for nursing to nurse the mind, body and spirit has been related to a case study. The role of rehabilitation and the different phases of rehabilitation have been explored and applied to a case study. Goal setting has been identified and discussed as a strategy that will support you to ensure that rehabilitation goals are achievable, promote the autonomy of the person and reflect their individual needs and aims. The concept of living with and beyond cancer has been introduced and related to rehabilitation.

Activities: brief outline answers

Activity 5.2: Critical thinking

Death from cancer – rehabilitation could be used at any point along the person's disease trajectory; however it could perhaps be most useful as the person's functional ability starts to decline and could focus on improving a person's physical independence as their disease progresses.

Death from organ failure – for people with organ failure rehabilitation could be particularly helpful following an exacerbation and could focus on promoting functional ability and enabling the person to maximise their independence.

Death from frailty and cognitive decline – in this trajectory rehabilitation could be used at any point along the continuum; it could be used to prevent or delay deterioration in a person's function and to improve their physical independence as their disease progresses.

Addressing a person's physical rehabilitation can impact positively on their emotional and psychological well being, improving their quality of life and emotional resilience in the face of living with dying.

Activity 5.3: Critical thinking

Preventative rehabilitation – at this point rehabilitation may focus on several areas of Chris's care: medication management (physical); you would need to ensure that Chris understands his medication, what it is for and when to take it/use it (harmony and mind). Increasing his understanding of his medication may alleviate some of Chris's anxieties about his health, e.g., talking him through what to do if he has an episode of chest pain (mind, healing and harmony). In addition ongoing monitoring of Chris's condition will inform the health care team of the efficacy of his treatment and its impact on his overall health and wellbeing (whole and harmony). Support Chris to increase his level of activity through encouraging him to take some form of regular exercise, explaining the benefits of this and exploring any concerns he may have (whole and harmony). These would be ongoing.

Restorative rehabilitation – the aim here is to return Chris to his previous level of activity, focusing on exercises to strengthen leg muscles and to develop his core strength (body). Teaching Chris some simple exercises to improve lung function and breathing techniques to use when breathless could also be considered and would reduce anxiety (body, mind and harmony). In addition acknowledging the psychological impact the diagnosis of COPD could have on Chris is also important, giving Chris time to talk and discuss any concerns he has (mind, healing and harmony). This would be time limited, ideally within 2/3 weeks so that Chris has a clear goal to aim for.

Supportive rehabilitation – at this point your aim will be to maximise Chris's functional capacity and maintain as much independence as possible (body), focusing on what he can still achieve (mind, spirit and healing). This may involve the use of adaptive equipment, e.g., walking stick/frame; in addition you would want to encourage Chris to continue with exercises to maintain the strength in his legs (body and harmony). Involvement of other members of the primary health care team would also be relevant, e.g., occupational therapist regarding energy saving aids (perching stool, commode) (harmony). The intervention of the members of the health care team may be time limited; however the interventions would be ongoing.

Palliative rehabilitation – involving Chris's carers in his rehabilitation would be important; they could undertake passive limb exercises and could encourage Chris to carry out some active limb exercises while they are getting him washed and dressed (body and harmony). Ensuring effective symptom control would also form part of Chris's rehabilitation, therefore providing information about when to take his lorazepam and how to reduce anxiety could contribute to improving Chris's quality of life (whole, harmony and healing). While Chris has expressed an interest to be cared for at home, it may be necessary to discuss alternative options with Chris, giving him the opportunity to remain in control of his situation (whole, harmony and healing).

Activity 5.4: Decision-making

At this point in her disease trajectory the main focus of Esther's rehabilitation is supportive. Due to her second stroke it is not likely that she will return to her previous level of function; however it is early on in her rehabilitation and restorative rehabilitation should not be discounted.

Mobility	
Specific	Able to transfer independently from bed to chair and back again
Measurable	Currently Esther needs the support of two members of staff to transfer; progress will be measurable as her reliance on staff reduces
Achievable	Esther has scored herself at 7; this indicates there is a good chance this goal will be achieved
Realistic	A score of 7 indicates this is a realistic goal for Esther to achieve as long as the timeframe is not too short
Timed	2 weeks would be a realistic timeframe for this goal to be achieved

It would be appropriate to include the following members of the multidisciplinary team:

- physiotherapist – for input regarding strengthening and mobility exercises, advice regarding safe manual handling;
- occupational therapist – for input regarding aids and adaptive equipment, e.g., chair raisers, walking aids;

- podiatrist – as Esther has type 2 diabetes her feet should be regularly inspected; a podiatrist could come and cut her toenails and ensure that there are no other foot issues that might affect her mobility;
- Esther's husband and son – including Esther's husband and son in this plan will mean that should Esther want to get in/out of bed when her family were present they would be able to assist her to do this safely and in line with her rehabilitation plan. Involving the family in the 'safer' hospital setting has the potential to increase their confidence in being able to support Esther when she returns home.

Returning to her involvement in the church lunch club:

This is a significantly broader and longer term goal; however it is an important goal for Esther as she has been involved in this club for quite some time and it plays an important role in her overall health and well being (whole and healing). It may not be possible to compile a SMART goal for this part of Esther's rehabilitation; instead it may be necessary to identify smaller goals that will go towards supporting her to achieve this longer term goal (whole, healing and harmony). For example, compiling a SMART goal in relation to her dysarthria (body and harmony), with support from a speech and language therapist, will increase her ability to participate in helping at the lunch club (healing). Reaching her goal in relation to her mobility (body) will mean that she is able to travel to the church and take part when she is there (whole). This longer term goal will require involvement of many members of the health care team: physiotherapist, occupational therapist, speech and language therapist, orthotist (adaptive equipment for mobility may be required, e.g., splints) and family members, especially if they are going to be required to take Esther to and from the lunch club.

Activity 5.5: Critical thinking

You may have listed some of the following though you may also have added some of your own.

Physical – scarring, weight loss/gain, incontinence, pain, neuropathy, dysarthria, dysphagia, stoma, facial/body disfigurement, amputation, pain during sex, erectile dysfunction, oral/dental problems, breathing difficulties, osteoporosis, hair loss, lymphoedema, nausea/vomiting, bowel or bladder adhesions, fistulas

Social and emotional – fear of their cancer recurring, reduced self-confidence, problems with their memory and/or concentration, financial worries, stress, depression, changed perspective on life, unable to return to work/education, difficulty in coping with changes to their physical self, which may impact on relationships

Further reading

Bennett, B., Breeze, J. and Neilson, T. (2014) Applying the recovery model to physical rehabilitation. *Nursing Standard*, 28 (23): 37–43.

The recovery model has been used in the field of mental health for over 20 years. This article explores the relationship between the recovery model and physical rehabilitation. This approach could be considered for those living with and beyond cancer.

Khan, N.F., Harrison, S., Rose, P.W., Ward, A. and Evans, J. (2012) Interpretation and acceptance of the term 'cancer survivor': a United Kingdom based qualitative study. *European Journal of Cancer Care*, 21: 177–186.

Tiberini, R. and Richardson, H. (2015) *Rehabilitative Palliative Care, Enabling People to Live Fully Until They Die, a Challenge for the 21st Century.* London: Hospice UK.

This report includes information about how to implement rehabilitation for people receiving palliative and end of life care. It includes practical tips and best practice examples.

Useful websites

www.hospiceuk.org/what-we-offer/clinical-and-care-support/rehabilitative-palliative-care

This link takes you to the main Hospice UK webpage for rehabilitative palliative care. It includes a range of resources relating to rehabilitation in palliative and end of life care, including resources to support the implementation and delivery of rehabilitation in palliative and end of life care.

www.macmillan.org.uk/about-us/health-professionals/programmes-and-services/consequences-of-treatment

These pages from the Macmillan Cancer Support website include information, guidance and advice on their consequences of treatment programme. The information can be used by health care professionals, people living with and beyond cancer and their families.

Chapter 6
Ethical issues in palliative and end of life care

Sherri Ogston-Tuck

NMC Standards for Pre-registration Nursing Education

This chapter will address the following competencies:

Domain 1: Professional values

1. All nurses must practise with confidence according to *The Code: Professional Standards of Practice and Behaviour for Nurses and Midwives* (NMC 2015), and within other recognised ethical and legal frameworks. They must be able to recognise and address ethical challenges relating to people's choices and decision making about their care, and act within the law to help them and their families and carers find acceptable solutions.

Domain 2: Communication and interpersonal skills

2. All nurses must use a range of communication skills and technologies to support person-centred care and enhance quality and safety. They must ensure people receive all the information they need in a language and manner that allows them to make informed choices and share decision making. They must recognise when language interpretation or other communication support is needed and know how to obtain it.

Domain 4: Leadership, management and team working

4. All nurses must be self-aware and recognise how their own values, principles and assumptions may affect their practice. They must maintain their own personal and professional development, learning from experience, through supervision, feedback, reflection and evaluation.

NMC Essential Skills Clusters

This chapter will address the following ESCs:

Cluster: Care, compassion and communication

3. People can trust the newly registered graduate nurse to respect them as individuals and strive to help them preserve their dignity at all times.

continued ... •

First progression point

1. Demonstrates respect for diversity and individual preferences, valuing differences, regardless of personal view.

Entry to the register

6. Acts autonomously to challenge situations or others when someone's dignity may be compromised.

4. People can trust a newly qualified graduate nurse to engage with them and their family or carers within their cultural environments in an acceptable and anti-discriminatory manner free from harassment and exploitation.

First progression point

3. Adopts a principled approach to care underpinned by *The Code* (NMC 2015).

Entry to the register

5. Is acceptant of differing cultural traditions, beliefs, UK legal frameworks and professional ethics when planning care with people and their families and carers.

Chapter aims

After reading this chapter you will be able to:

• understand the theories and principles of medical and health care ethics;
• consider your role in recognising ethical and legal challenges relating to palliative and end of life care;
• reflect on your own values and thoughts about people's choices and decision making about their care at end of life and explore these in terms of your role as a nurse;
• consider the ethical debate on research with patients at the end of life and in palliative care.

Introduction

Maria wanted to be a nurse for as long as she could remember ... she believed that she would be a good nurse. But five years on since her qualification, Maria has started to question this. 'Am I a good nurse? I don't feel like I am making a difference ...'

Questioning whether someone is a good nurse may be helpful in understanding what ethics means in nursing practice. Ethics in itself is about 'what is good', in contrast to 'what is right'. However it is not as simple as debating the nature of good nursing – this would not make Maria a 'good' nurse. Understanding how people become good nurses will help to underpin our understanding of ethics in nursing, and in health care practice.

Ethics is not something separate from patient care that you only think about occasionally (Hawley 2007). The very nature of ethics requires you to reflect on your actions, to consider reasons for those actions and outcomes. This requires consideration of anticipated outcomes, and more importantly, the decisions made and consequences of your actions. Serious engagement in ethics highlights some of the tensions between nursing as an ethical role and as a professional, legal or institutional role (Tingle and Cribb 2007). Health care is becoming increasingly more technically advanced. New medicines, treatment options and surgical procedures are available where they were not before. Difficult decisions are being made where once there would have been no decision to make, because the option simply was not there. People are undergoing more radical treatment that extends the quantity of their life, but not necessarily its quality. For patients with a terminal diagnosis, it is important that they are involved in the decision-making process and have the ability to steer the direction of their treatment. Strategies like advance care planning (ACP) allow patients to participate in this process actively and decide what treatment they may or may not wish to have in the future. These changes have increased and heightened the importance of nursing ethics that emphasises professional accountability, policy, frameworks and guidelines, and personal responsibility. Ethics asks you to consider what is right and wrong, and challenges you to reflect on your own belief systems. This chapter will support you in your ability to apply an ethical framework to your clinical practice. It will encourage you to consider the ethical issues that are evident in palliative and end of life care.

What is ethics?

Your professional role demands that you consider the ethical implications of decisions made in your day-to-day practice. Ethics in clinical practice can be regarded as quality care (Bishop and Scudder 2001), where the ethical ideal of caring requires you to be culturally sensitive and competent (Hawley 2007). Beliefs are certain principles which we argue should be followed by other people, and which we use as a standard for our own personal behaviour. These everyday ethical reflections and judgements are important.

In nursing and health care practice ethics is rarely approached as a separate entity from both legal and professional dimensions. Together, they help you to question what is good (ethical dimension) and what is right (legal dimension) and in making decisions and taking action (professional dimension) for patients in your care. It is from the outcome of these, and indeed the role of the nurse, that ethics may be understood more clearly. As a nurse, your goal is to promote health and to prevent harm, and to some extent perhaps this is what Maria is questioning when she asks herself whether she is a good nurse.

The values that shape nursing practice reflect the nature of the nurse–patient relationship and elicit ideas such as empowerment, partnership and advocacy. Nursing ethics involves making decisions and value judgements about nursing care and 'what is good nursing'.

At the centre of this is patient care, but what are the aims of care? What you value in nursing care reflects your professional role to deliver good care, and the decisions you make to provide safe and effective care and promote health and wellbeing. The values built into this and your delivery of care underpins ethics, and the principles of ethics. This is about values, choice and judgements. Many of the key ethical issues nurses face stem from what nurses perceive their role to be – that of a good nurse – and of the care they give: good care.

The term ethics is used broadly in the context of our values and morals: what we perceive to be good or bad, right or wrong. It also encompasses professionalism – 'professional ethics'. According to Beauchamp and Childress (2009) ethics is a generic term covering several different ways of examining and understanding the 'moral life'. Seeking to 'act ethically' or to 'be ethical' requires first recognising that a moral situation exists. A moral situation forces you to think about what you would want for yourself, how you would want to be treated and what you value as an individual, and then to extend this to your patients. An ethical issue can arise from any of the following:

- when you have to judge what is right or wrong;
- choosing between options;
- deciding whether to do something or do nothing;
- asking yourself: should I or shouldn't I?;
- weighing up the potential impact of your decisions or actions;
- a dilemma – making a difficult choice.

Your understanding of the concepts of right and wrong is inherent, where you consciously have a grasp of the core dimensions of morality: not to lie; not to steal; to respect others; not to kill or cause harm to innocent persons. Therefore 'common morality' is a concept shared by all people, who are committed to morality. In ethics, this gives rise to rules of obligations, which are moral characteristics or virtues.

Virtues in ethics are questions about your character – qualities of character; admirable or desirable dispositions. This is important in nursing ethics, and helps to answer what it is that makes you a 'good nurse'.

Activity 6.1   *Reflection*

Think for a moment about how you would describe yourself. What morals or virtues do you hold?

Of the list of virtues below, choose those that you feel are necessary for nursing:

Honesty   Integrity   Truthfulness   Loyalty   Patience   Humility

Courage   Resilience

Would you add anything to this list?

Brief answers to all activities are given at the end of the chapter, unless otherwise indicated.

In completing Activity 6.1 it is likely that the words you used to describe yourself were also reflected in the morals/virtues you felt were necessary for nursing. This allows you to see that the morals you hold as a person have the potential to influence how you are as a nurse, highlighting the potential for dilemmas to occur.

What is an ethical dilemma?

Ethical issues in health care are defined as those phenomena or behaviours that have the potential to become a problem (Hawley 2007). Ethical problems are those incidents or situations that have arisen from a moral or ethical issue and which are vitally important in the life of the patient. The following are examples of questions that raise intrinsic philosophical matters to do with the nature and value of life:

- Is it right that someone should be left to die in pain, without choice, because it is a fundamental human right to life?
- Is it wrong to end life where there is suffering and futility of life?

In health care, ethics refers to a wide range of practice situations. There are few decisions, actions or omissions that do not have an ethical dimension (Beauchamp and Childress 2009). It is impossible to treat these issues seriously without some consideration of moral and ethical questioning. Doing this generates awareness of your own limitations. However, being 'philosophically skilled' does not necessarily mean being a good person but it does mean taking an interest in your character as well as your actions (Tingle and Cribb 2007).

It is possible – sometimes all too easy – not to do what you regard as the right thing. Ethics in health care is about doing the right thing in a certain situation and being a certain kind of person in that situation (Gallagher and Hodge 2012). There are some ethical 'rules' that can be applied to your practice. These underpin your professional role, morals, conscience and virtues:

- veracity – truth telling, informed consent, respect for autonomy;
- privacy – a person's right to remain private, not to disclose information;
- confidentiality – only sharing private information on a 'need to know' basis;
- fidelity – loyalty, maintaining the duty to care for all, no matter who they are or what they may have done.

Activity 6.2   *Reflection*

Consider the list of ethical rules above. Which of these do you possess as a virtue?

You may have found that some of the ethical rules you said you possess in Activity 6.2 mirror those qualities that you listed in Activity 6.1. These underlying virtues and rules underpin your response to specific situations. To support you in your decision making we will now discuss some of the theories used in ethics.

Theories in ethics

Before considering theories of ethics and their differences there are some other aspects of ethics that need to be considered. Ethics has to do with 'how people act' and 'how people behave' and as a starting point can be broadly separated into *consequentialism*, taking the consequences of your actions into consideration, and *deontology*, basing your actions on a set of principles or duties.

Normative ethics is concerned with what people 'should or ought to do' and how they should live. Non-normative ethics (or *descriptive ethics*) seeks to establish the facts of a situation, not what ought to be done. It is a form of inquiry to answer the question of moral norms (normative ethics), whereas in non-normative ethics this aims to investigate the facts of moral conduct of how people reason or act (Beauchamp and Childress 2009). For example, determining which moral norms and attitudes are expressed in professional practice. In nursing this would be derived from your professional code of conduct or determined from the organisational mission statement or policy. The scenario below illustrates how both normative and non-normative ethics are evident in your clinical practice.

Scenario

Staff nurse Susan is caring for Bill who was admitted to the ward with chronic liver failure. He is unsteady on his feet, often confused and unable to care for himself alone at home. Bill is 78, and a 'larger than life' character as described by his family and friends. He has been a heavy drinker for many years. Bill's wife died more than 25 years ago and his family recognises that part of coping with bereavement has been heavier drinking and a carefree lifestyle. Bill is not coping well and is frustrated, mainly by his limited mobility and reliance on carers. Bill often lashes out and refuses help. He shouts at the nurses and tells them he can take care of himself and is going home. Susan wants to be a good nurse and tries to provide the care Bill needs, helping him with his washing, with feeding and offering to shave and tidy his beard. She knows that Bill wants to be independent and she is struggling to balance helping him without taking his independence away.

In this situation normative ethics is evident in that Bill does not feel that his refusal of help is causing him ill health and he does not feel that he needs to be 'taken care of'. He refuses to accept he needs to be 'in care' and does not understand that at home alone he would be putting himself at risk of a fall or worse. Susan is approaching this from a non-normative ethics perspective. She knows what the facts of the situation are – a risk of falling, and not eating or caring for himself would put Bill at unnecessary risk. She wants to help Bill and prevent undue harm.

Empirical ethics can be used to support your nursing practice. Generally, empirical ethics involves data collection from questions, focus groups or observations about people and their actions, thoughts, feelings and behaviours. Empirical ethics informs your practice and, in many ways, highlights the importance and relevance of research and evidence-based practice. To explore this theory let us develop the scenario with Susan and Bill further.

Activity 6.3	*Critical thinking*

A recent study on liver cirrhosis and advancing liver failure placed patients at greater risk of malnutrition, with higher incidences of confusion as the disease progressed. This was largely due to the liver's inability to metabolise drugs and break down toxins. Although the damage to the liver cannot be repaired, a healthy diet and support with orientation and mobility can help patients in coping with their activities of daily living.

How does this help Susan and her dilemma in caring for Bill?

Utilitarianism

Utilitarianism is often referred to as a consequentialist-based theory. This is because it involves weighing up the consequences of an action. It holds that actions are right or wrong according to the balance of their good or bad consequences. This theory concentrates on the value of wellbeing or intrinsic good, such as happiness and pleasure, freedom and health, welfare and preference satisfaction. This can be illustrated in the scenario above. It could be considered that Bill's refusal of care and wanting to go home provides him with comfort and independence. This outweighs the bad consequences of being in a place that he does not want to be. For Bill, the surroundings and routines are unfamiliar, which heightens his hostility and frustration. His confusion is exacerbated by this and he sees the carers only as an interference and a trigger for his outbursts. Susan's dilemma is in recognising this and trying to balance the good and bad consequences of Bill's behaviour, supporting him to familiarise himself with his new environment and to see the help as less intrusive. Her duty of care is not to harm Bill and it would be unlawful for Susan to physically stop Bill from leaving. However she is obligated to provide him with a safe environment. It is important that she tries to reassure Bill and, when he is less confused, tries to explain to him that she is there to help. He needs to be enabled to see the benefit of the care and assistance with eating and washing. It is equally important that Bill is able to make autonomous decisions for himself. This may be facilitated by offering choice and timing of, for example, his washing or activities of daily living. It would be unethical for Susan not to consider both sides of this dilemma, but she cannot stop Bill from exercising his own free will and choice. The obligation in this scenario is to respect Bill and his decisions; this is the moral dilemma Susan faces. With utilitarianism it is the end or consequences that are important and dictate whether the action is ethical. It is measured in a positive or negative relation to good or happiness and pain or unhappiness (time is immaterial).

Kantianism

Kantian ethics (Immanuel Kant, 1724–1804, German philosopher) or deontological theory, is modelled on 'moral worth' and 'moral acceptability'. It can be described as duty-based or an obligation. In health care this obligation would include respect for individuals. In the scenario above, you can see how Susan has an ethical dilemma, in trying to help Bill make decisions for his self-care and to ensure he is safe and free of harm. Her duty of care is not to harm Bill however difficult this may be. Kant's theory of duty involves holding some features or actions as good in themselves, regardless of their consequences. One of Kant's most important claims is that the moral worth of an individual's action depends exclusively on the moral acceptability of the rule (or 'maxim'). The rule provides a moral reason that justifies the action (Beauchamp and Childress 2009).

Activity 6.4   *Decision-making*

Using the information in the scenario above, can you identify the moral reasoning that justifies Susan's actions? If possible, share your ideas with a colleague and see whether you agree.

Rights theory or 'liberal individualism'

Rights theory (Beauchamp and Childress 2009) employs the language of rights – civil, political and legal rights – in protecting individuals. Rights-based ethical theory makes claims that are justified; this is a basis for both international and national frameworks in ethical practice. It offers some positive rights – this requires something of others – and some negative rights – this requires that people are left alone without interference. However, rights are not absolute, even the right to life (as evidenced by common moral judgements such as killing in war). Therefore it is necessary to balance claims and distinguish between a violation of a right (an unjustified action against a right) and an infringement of a right (a justified action overriding a right) (Nielson (1993), cited in Beauchamp and Childress (2009)). Returning to the scenario above, preventing Bill from leaving hospital may be a violation of his right to make choices, whether good or bad, for himself. But if the risk is great and goes against Susan's obligation to prevent harm, this infringement may be justified.

Communitarianism

This theory holds communal values such as the common good, social goals, traditional practices and cooperative virtues, all of which are fundamental in ethics. Virtues-based ethics offers the theoretical approach that focuses on character and ethical qualities or those dispositions of health care professionals.

Activity 6.5   *Critical thinking*

List the virtues Susan will need to demonstrate when caring for Bill.

You may have identified Susan must demonstrate respect and compassion for Bill. These virtues reflect the professional values of nurses as described in *The Code* (NMC 2015). Many ethical theories have moral implications, in that one has to think through the ethical implications of one's decisions and actions. As a result of these different ways of thinking and doing, conflict exists. An ethical framework can support you in working your way through these conflicts.

Ethical frameworks

Beauchamp and Childress's (2009) principles of biomedical ethics ('the principalist approach') address four key moral principles: autonomy, beneficence, non-maleficence and justice. They provide a broad framework that can be used for ethical deliberation and discussion, most notably in health care practice. The principles consider deciding how to act (Tingle and Cribb 2007), where health care professionals ought to respect autonomy and avoid harm, where possible benefit the patient and consider (fairly) the interests of all those affected. Although this framework has been highly criticised as being too simplistic and too mechanical, it offers a critical and thoughtful approach to support you in your ethical decision making. It is important to note, however, that *not all* ethical thinking can be reduced to a few key words or that four principles will provide a quick and easy method for you to use when approaching ethical dilemmas. Rather, the principalist approach provides a reminder of key dimensions of ethical thinking (Tingle and Cribb 2007).

Autonomy

The principle of autonomy recognises the rights of individuals to self-determination. It acknowledges individuals' rights to hold views, make choices and take actions based on their personal values and beliefs (Beauchamp and Childress 2009). Autonomy is an important social value in terms of what is important to the patient, rather than to you as a nurse and to other health care professionals. It is also an indicator of what health means to a patient. Individuals can experience loss of autonomy if they are unwell and no longer able to participate in their life in the way they once did. We can see this in Bill's case. Overall, having autonomy can be a general indicator of health. For you respecting autonomy involves supporting rules and obligations to tell the truth, respect for privacy and maintaining confidentiality (Beauchamp and Childress 2009). Key components of this principle require you to respect patients' rights to make their own decisions, to teach people to be able to make their own choices and to support this without force or coercion. An important outcome of this principle is informed consent (see Chapter 8) and it is also the basis for advance decision to refuse treatment decisions.

Activity 6.6   *Critical thinking*

Adeeba is 72 and has a complex chronic respiratory condition. A stroke has left her with weakness in her right side and reduced mobility. Adeeba is on continuous home oxygen therapy and uses a CPAP (continuous positive airway pressure) device when she is sleeping.

---

continued ... •

Adeeba's main carer is her husband and for the past two years she has been restricted to her bed and has had an indwelling urinary catheter for the last six months. Adeeba sleeps most of the day. She does not eat the meals her husband prepares and often refuses to take her medication. She tells her husband every day this is no life and she just wants to die.

The district nurses visit Adeeba twice daily. On this occasion Stella, the visiting nurse, finds Adeeba quite poorly. Her heart rate is very low (40 bpm) and she is struggling to breathe. Her lips are cyanotic even with oxygen on (her respiratory rate is 28 bpm and her SPAO2 is 88 per cent). Stella tells Adeeba she needs to go to hospital but she refuses. She wants to stay at home.

Consider the following questions:

- How will Stella respect Adeeba's autonomy?
- What should she do?

You may have identified that Stella would need to provide Adeeba with enough information for her to be able to make an informed decision about her treatment. You may have recognised that Adeeba's autonomy is already compromised, and that this could impact on her legal competence to refuse treatment (see Chapter 8). An autonomous decision does not have to be the 'correct' decision, otherwise individual needs and values would not be respected. Rather, an autonomous decision is one that is an informed decision.

Non-maleficence

The principle of non-maleficence is embodied by the main consideration to 'do no harm'. You should not cause pain or suffering; you should not incapacitate or cause offence; you should not deprive people; you should not kill.

It is more important not to harm your patients than to do them good. For health care professionals, this influences every intervention, treatment and decision that is made for patients. It is believed that these will do good; however, first you need to consider whether they do no harm, or acceptable levels of harm. Non-maleficence underpins evidence-based practice (as does the principle of beneficence – doing good). This relates to issues of consent, and understanding whether treatment is likely to be harmful. The patient should understand the risks and benefits, and that the likely benefits outweigh the likely risks. Unfortunately this principle is not absolute, and must also be balanced against the principle of beneficence.

| Activity 6.7 | *Critical thinking* |

Adeeba's husband insists that the ambulance takes her to hospital. He sees his wife struggling to breathe and is worried. Stella rings 999. Adeeba is distressed but hasn't the strength to argue with her husband.

Remember, this principle requires you to do no harm to your patient. Ask yourself the following questions:

- Would the patient be harmed by the treatment, i.e., by forcibly restraining her on the ambulance trolley? How will Adeeba be affected if she is not taken to hospital now for treatment?
- Would it be impractical for the ambulance to take her to the hospital if Adeeba does not want to go? And if so, which course of action would result in the greatest harm?
- Are there any alternatives?

Activity 6.7 highlights the dilemmas faced by both patients and health care professionals. In this scenario they both know that the short term outcome is that without emergency treatment Adeeba will likely collapse as her breathing becomes more laboured; this could lead to respiratory arrest and she may die. It could be argued that it is selfish or unfair for Adeeba's husband to insist she go to hospital when Adeeba does not want to.

Beneficence

The principle of beneficence is one of the core values of health care ethics and is considered in relation to non-maleficence and preventing harm where you 'ought to do good'. It requires weighing up what it means to do good as opposed to what will bring about harm or wrong (Gallagher and Hodge 2012). The term beneficence refers to actions that promote the wellbeing of others, such as creating a safe and supportive environment and helping people in crisis. Our actions must aim to 'benefit' people – their health, welfare, comfort and wellbeing, improving a person's potential and quality of life.

Importantly, 'benefit' should be defined by the individuals themselves. It is not what you think that is important. In the medical context, this means taking actions that serve the best interests of patients. This means acting on behalf of vulnerable people, to protect their rights and prevent them from harm. However, uncertainty surrounds the precise definition of which practices do in fact help patients. This is true of end of life care and quality of life issues.

Activity 6.8	Critical thinking

Ivan is 54, in a hospice, and dying of terminal cancer. Ivan has actively planned his death and does not want his partner to worry. Ivan has been prescribed morphine to help alleviate his pain and to keep him comfortable. However, at the same time, the side-effects of the potent opioid analgesic are causing Ivan to feel nauseated, he is often vomiting and he is very drowsy. Ivan's partner Ewan is concerned that he is still suffering. He knows that Ivan did not want this.

continued ... •

Ivan is now refusing any further treatment.

Remember, this principle requires you to act to benefit the patient. It may also clash with the principle of respect for autonomy when the patient makes a decision that the health care professional does not think will benefit the patient – is not in the patient's 'best interests'. Now ask yourself the following questions:

- How can the balance to benefit Ivan while minimising the harmful side-effects of treatment be achieved?
- Is there a benefit to having the patient's autonomy overridden?
- Have both the long term and short term effects been considered? Without treatment, will Ivan suffer more? Would stopping treatment hasten his death or prolong his pain and suffering?

The scenario in Activity 6.8 poses a difficult dilemma. It would be helpful if you were aware of an advance decision to refuse treatment (ADRT) (see Chapter 8 for further information) that tells you Ivan's wishes for his end of life care. Although he has made plans, it is not known how this has been communicated. It is also important that his family are aware of his wishes, so Ivan's autonomy is respected and decisions are made in his best interests, which may well be to die with dignity, without pain and without suffering. The benefits of acting beneficently would need to be weighed against the benefits of failing to respect Ivan's autonomy. From a legal point of view the wishes of a competent adult patient cannot be overridden in their best interests.

Justice

The principle of justice is about you treating people fairly and not favouring some individuals or groups over others. You should act in a non-discriminatory or non-prejudicial way. It is also about what is fair and just in the distribution of limited health resources, and the decision as to who gets what treatment. Underlying this principle is equality, which is both challenging and often difficult to grasp in practice. It is based on need, effort, contribution and management. Everyone and everything has an equal share and this principle underpins respect for people's rights and respect for the law.

Case study

If we revisit the scenario with Adeeba, her long term condition is pulmonary hypertension and 5 years ago, when the cardiac specialists told her there was little hope of reversing her condition, she participated in a drug trial. Adeeba responded favourably to the treatment which cost over £1000 a month. However, any further improvement is unlikely and her condition has now plateaued. The specialists have told her she will not get any better, though she may not get any worse. The drug maintains the pressure in her pulmonary artery and without it she would most certainly die.

The expensive treatment is Adeeba's only hope of living.

Is the issue of cost relevant? Or is the potential benefit for the individual? The difficulty in this decision is the provision of a very expensive life-saving/life-prolonging drug and the quality and futility of life. Is it fair that this treatment is continued at such a cost when there is little improvement expected or where others could benefit from this more so than Adeeba?

What is fair and just is very difficult to determine in this case study, with both cost and the greater good being contributing factors. In some cases the cost of treatment has to be the trade-off, where other treatment options are available and cheaper. This will override what is fair versus what is just.

Here the benefit of treatment has been favoured as fair and just – and the cost is not relevant.

Adeeba has said on numerous occasions that this life is not worth living ... she recognises that her quality of life has deteriorated. She has no appetite, spends most days in bed and tells her husband to stop giving her the medication. She refuses to eat anything.

Adeeba's husband consults with her doctor, who tells her if she stops the medication her heart will stop in less than 48 hours and she would die.

How does this influence your ethical decision making?

By applying the four principles approach, it can help with ethical dilemmas and decision making. The process requires you to stand back, draw on reflection, engage in discussion and debate. This will provide you with a practical framework. It is not formulaic and although this approach has its limitations (Gallagher and Hodge 2012), it can be very helpful in structuring how you think through the ethical problems that underpin your professional actions.

Activity 6.9   *Critical thinking*

Paul is 70 and has had a serious fall outside his home. He was left lying on the pavement for two hours before his neighbour found him. Paul is taken to hospital, with a deep laceration on his forehead and a compound fracture of his humerus.

Routine blood work is done and X-rays of the fracture. Some of the blood tests show changes in Paul's renal function. He has had hypertension for years but stopped taking his mediations because he did not like how they made him feel. Paul often experiences dizziness and headaches. Further investigations and blood tests confirm prostate cancer.

Paul's daughter Rose has been worried about him and insisted that he be more careful at home; he is unsteady on his feet at the best of times. Paul does not want her to be

continued ...

informed of this – he tells you 'Please don't tell Rose, it will only worry her ... Please, I don't want her to know'.

Rose arrives on the ward and asks you how he is; she tells you that he is keeping something from her.

Now answer the following questions:

- What does it mean to respect the patient's autonomy?
- What harm, if any, might result from telling Rose of his diagnosis?
- What is the most just response in this situation?

High-quality patient care

When caring for patients receiving palliative and end of life care it is important that you recognise relatives need to be assured that high-quality care will be delivered and that the wishes of the patient will be respected (Andershed 2006). The importance of nurses and other health care professionals developing a trusting relationship with an open, positive attitude has been identified as an important factor in palliative and end of life care. In addition, being sensitive to the needs of relatives for information and education through effective communication has been recognised (Oberle and Hughes 2001; Andershed 2006). Relatives felt supported and experienced peace of mind when they knew that nurses and other health care professionals were acting in their dying loved one's best interest (Oberle and Hughes 2001; Gott et al. 2004).

Activity 6.10   *Evidence-based practice*

Henry is 54. He was admitted to hospital five days ago with pneumonia. He has been receiving treatment for cancer for two years and only just a few months ago felt that that he was getting stronger and better. Henry's condition is now deteriorating. He is distressed and semiconscious. His breathing is laboured, even with oxygen being administered. He moans audibly on expiration, suggesting he is in a great deal of pain and discomfort. Henry's relatives have asked the staff about his breathing and are also worried that he is in pain. The health care team discusses Henry's situation and an agreement is reached, but this is not supported by all staff. Henry will be prescribed morphine to control the pain. Some staff are concerned this may compromise his already weak respiratory system. Others feel that, while morphine may cause respiratory depression, the effect of the drug will relax Henry's respiratory muscles and he will not have to work as hard to breathe and therefore he will have less pain.

Now consider the following questions and apply the ethical principles to your decision making:

- Are staff correct in their assumption that morphine will compromise the already weakened respiratory system? If so, why? If not, why not?
- Do you think this is the right treatment for Henry? If so, why? If not, why not?
- What information would you provide to Henry's family and how?

There may not be a right or wrong answer for the questions in Activity 6.10. However, one thing is certain: the nurse has an important role in this situation.

Research in end of life and palliative care

Currently there is ongoing debate in terms of the use and value of research where patients at the end of life and in palliative care are the research participants. Addington-Hall (2007) argues that there is a poor developed research base in palliative care; one of the reasons for this is the lack of research and the variable quality undertaken. The main factor for this is the difficulty in conducting research with the very ill and bereaved. The debate surrounding the ethics of researching end of life situations raises key issues such as vulnerability, consent, gate keeping, inclusion and research culture (Duke and Bennett 2010). Duke and Bennett further observed that while there was recognition of the importance of dignity, rights and safety of research participants, less attention was given to the needs and rights of researchers and their responsibility in dissemination.

The problems associated with including people who are dying and/or close to death in research encompasses the ethics of involving people at such a 'difficult stage' of their life and dealing with highly sensitive material. The very nature of this group of patients as participants poses ethical research issues and certain dilemmas because of the involvement of life threatening illnesses that have an unpredictable disease trajectory (Lee and Kristjanson 2003). This makes participation in, for example, longitudinal studies almost impossible. Furthermore, the illnesses are often distressingly complex in terms of their treatment, e.g., where high doses of medicine are needed to relieve symptoms – these can impair mental competence, making it difficult to consistently participate. Participation may be impeded due to reasons related to the illness, the way it can fluctuate, or other conditions that affect communication (Seymour et al. 2005). The needs of family members must also be considered, as they may find it hard to be involved in research because of the burden of care giving, fatigue and the emotional challenges associated with grief and loss (Gysels et al. 2013). Despite this, however, it is important that these individuals are given a 'voice' and the opportunity to participate (Clark 2003). In debating this dilemma, denying participation may be denying an opportunity to participate in research because of an unjustly paternalistic attitude (Gysels et al. 2012). Therefore one must consider the participants' sense of wanting to contribute to a greater community good. Others may argue participation may lead to neglect of their care and illness experience. An accurate attempt to balance the magnitude and probability of harm with the magnitude and probability of the benefit is necessary, first and foremost. This requires a thorough understanding of the nature and purpose of the research.

If research aims to create new knowledge through original investigations then one can argue the clear benefit of research – but it must be worthwhile and necessary. The value of knowledge gained should outweigh the potential disruption or inconvenience caused to those involved. In qualitative approaches a benefit could be distinguished as the very 'value in the participants' involvement' (Gysels et al. 2013). This can provide in-depth accounts of their own experience and the very circumstances that create them. This highlights that research is underpinned by key ethical principles:

1. That research must be justified.
2. That participation in research must be voluntary.
3. That confidentiality must be ensured.
4. That participants and the researcher(s) should not come to any harm during the research.

- The principle of autonomy is the respect of persons, and in research this informs the foundation of the participant's right to informed consent (see Chapter 8), to privacy and confidentiality. It involves respecting the participant's right to choose freely (free from pressure or coercion). The participant must be informed of the nature and purpose of the research. This includes any potential benefits, risks, and obligations of inconvenience associated with the research.
- It is important to note that only patients who are mentally competent to make such a decision can give informed consent (see Chapter 8). However this is a particular challenge in palliative care research because this patient group frequently experiences fluctuating cognitive ability, fatigue and depression, all of which can impact upon the process of consent. This is increasingly challenging in qualitative investigations, where the researcher negotiates the consent and then renegotiates the consent as unforeseen circumstances arise. The participant is part of the decision making as the study unfolds. However, when research takes place over a period of time, the participant's health may deteriorate, they may be in the last stages of dying and they may no longer be able to communicate. The person may have given their consent at the onset; however it is questionable whether this consent remains valid as their condition changes (Lawson 2001).
- The duty of the researcher(s) is not to inflict harm and to promote good. Therefore researchers have a duty to minimise risk and maximise benefits to participants. Research in palliative care is usually designed to improve the patients' or families' quality of life. This implies the principle of beneficence, to do the best for the patients and families. Participants ought to be treated fairly and in terms of research the protection of patients (as participants) from incompetence is fundamental.

In end of life care and palliative care research, it is important to consider where the duty of care (not to harm) versus duty to advance knowledge rests; the research imperative versus therapeutic imperative. At all times the therapeutic operative must take precedence over the research imperative. Ethical guidelines are not necessarily different for palliative care research but there are specific considerations for this population – patient vulnerability; treatment allocation; and gaining consent. This may mean that the way in which the benefits and burdens are distributed are justified in research but may require additional ethical demands on the research design and the methodology. Fair access to research treatments is an expectation of the justice principle, e.g., random selection of participants.

Activity 6.11   *Communication and decision-making*

- Recall Adeeba, who agreed to participate in a drug trial for the treatment of pulmonary hypertension. As her condition plateaued, Adeeba's cognitive function altered. Daily observations and her weight were required that fed into a database along with a record of any associated symptoms and/or side-effects. However some days Adeeba was less aware and not always compliant to the regimen.
- In terms of Adeeba's comprehension of the information and consent to participate, how might this impact upon the research trial? Is it ethical to continue?

As Activity 6.11 will have identified, in research there exists ethical issues and ethical acceptability, certainly in end of life care and palliative care. Participation is voluntary, and importantly, it is an invitation to participate rather than an expectation to participate. Recall the utilitarian and deontological perspective in ethics, where the utilitarian approach is for the greatest good for the greatest number. In terms of research the good of a project is defined by the consequences of the results. However, each researcher may have a different idea about what is good. The deontological perspective proposes an absolute moral imperative. In research deception in experiments is never justified – no matter what. Although some deontologists are more flexible making a distinction between harm and good, harm can be compensated for but wrongs cannot.

Chapter summary

Professional behaviour and standards of care underpin your role as a nurse and the care you deliver professionally, legally and morally. Importantly, reflecting on your own personal beliefs and values has an impact on your clinical and ethical decision making. This is of particular relevance in everyday practice, but even more significant in end of life care, where decision making is not as simple or straightforward. The use of ethical principles and frameworks can help to guide your decision making, and remind you where, and how, your own values and virtues can influence decisions made, hopefully for the better. However, achieving individual ethical integrity in life is difficult (Tschudin 2003, cited in Benjamin and Curtis 2011). In clinical practice, this needs to be inclusive of the multidisciplinary team, open communication and planning individual patient care. When you are faced with ethical dilemmas, adopting an ethical framework and reflective approach emphasises the importance of patient autonomy and choice in end of life care. Underpinning your ethical practice is the awareness of both your professional and legal obligations, to do good and not harm. The decisions you make should, and will, reflect your morals and values, because as nurses, as human beings, these are intrinsic to not only how you care, but also why you care.

Activities: brief outline answers

Activity 6.1: Reflection

You can describe yourself both as a person and as a nurse. Your morals and virtues are those characteristics that are unique to you; they are also those attributes that you possess in your professional role as a nurse. The virtues necessary for a nurse would include all of these: honesty, integrity, truthfulness, loyalty, patience, humility, courage and resilience. In addition you should be: compassionate, caring, competent, skilled, knowledgeable, kind, empathetic, insightful, open and honest, lawful, considerate, non-discriminatory, respectful, supportive, attentive, aware, facilitative, cooperative and impartial. These attributes and list of virtues reflect the NMC *Code* (2015).

Activity 6.2: Reflection

Veracity, privacy, confidentiality and fidelity are all essential virtues, reflecting those attributes that are essential for nursing and the standards of care and professional behaviour and attitude recommended by the NMC (2015).

Activity 6.3: Critical thinking

Susan can use this empirical data as evidence to inform the information she shares with Bill to help with his diet and orientation. This reflects the importance of how evidence is used in your practice. In this situation it can offload the judgement Susan may place on Bill and, with the evidence or statistics being presented, can help inform Susan and convey that she is trying to help Bill and in turn this may also sway his own decision making and autonomy.

Activity 6.4: Decision-making

For Susan the obligation here is to respect the individual: but this is the moral dilemma she faces. Although Susan has a professional duty and obligation to prevent harm, the infringement here may not be justified; Bill is able to make decisions for himself, whether you agree or not. Susan would need to be supported by her team and colleagues. She needs to ensure she has documented any discussion with Bill and the decisions about his self-care. However the worry and concern here is that Bill cannot care for himself at home alone and would be at greater risk. In some instances, where patients do not have the capacity to understand the risks this would pose, an assessment would be necessary to safeguard them and ensure that the decisions are not disproportionate to their autonomy and best interests. But safety remains paramount.

Activity 6.5: Critical thinking

Susan has demonstrated many of the virtues listed. She is respectful and non-judgemental; she is honest and acts with compassion and integrity. She also draws on her knowledge and skill and works collaboratively with her team and tries to make decisions that are in Bill's best interests.

Activity 6.6: Critical thinking

Unless determined otherwise, if Adeeba is able to make decisions for herself, her autonomy must be respected and upheld. A non-judgemental and empathetic approach is needed whilst also ensuring that Adeeba has all the relevant information to make her decisions. If Adeeba has the capacity to do this, and even if her nurse feels this is an unwise decision, it is Adeeba's to make. If Adeeba's capacity is in question it is not the nurse alone who would seek to challenge or determine this. Adeeba needs to understand the risks and benefits of further treatment that may only be obtained if she goes to hospital. It is important for her to understand that her breathing may improve and this may not be permanent. An informed decision to refuse to go to hospital must be clearly documented and communicated with the health care team and any alternative treatment discussed with Adeeba. Stella's dilemma here is making a decision in Adeeba's best interests and trying to determine whether the benefit of going to hospital would outweigh the risk of not going.

Activity 6.7: Critical thinking

Forcing treatment would be conceived as harmful and forcibly restraining Adeeba in order to get her into the ambulance would be unlawful. This would have an impact on the trust between Adeeba and Stella, and indeed Adeeba's husband (and the ambulance crew). Any alternative treatments or therapies must be considered and the limitations of these being delivered in the home recognised. It is likely that interventions needed to improve her breathing can only be provided if she goes to the local hospital. This information needs to be explained clearly to Adeeba. However, Stella (and the ambulance crew) have an obligation to ensure both the risks and benefits of any alternatives, reckoning that hospitalisation is in Adeeba's best interests. Respecting the patient's wishes in this instance is difficult. Although Adeeba's autonomy must be respected, her decision making and capacity to do this may be impaired. Adeeba's husband, as her next of kin, can insist she go to hospital, but it is Adeeba's decisions (and her capacity to make them) that pose the dilemma here. Without an ADRT this is impossible to determine. If the ambulance is called as the situation escalates to an emergency this may indeed prevail over Adeeba's decision to refuse to go to the hospital.

Activity 6.8: Critical thinking

To act in a way that benefits Ivan, it is necessary to first respect his autonomy and his wishes. Striking a balance between benefit and harm is not easy, and this is where the clash in respecting Ivan's choice for himself is the challenge. It is essential to keep Ivan comfortable and pain free; and it is equally important to manage the side-effects of the pain relief in his best interests. One could argue there is no benefit to overriding Ivan's autonomy and to continue treatment. In the short term, he is *less likely* to suffer, but without adequate pain relief, more suffering is likely.

Activity 6.9: Critical thinking

Patient autonomy is about what is important to the patient. Therefore it is necessary to respect Paul's wishes and disclosure of confidential information, even to his daughter. The nurse caring for Paul must respect his autonomy and support his decision for his daughter not to be told his diagnosis. Even if there is an underlying obligation to tell Paul's daughter, this truth would not be respectful of Paul's wishes or for his privacy and confidentiality. Paul has the right to make his own decisions and own choices here, however difficult these might be for the nurse. At the moment the health care professionals have a duty of care to Paul, to respect his wishes and to keep his daughter informed of the treatment and care. Beyond this and disclosure of his diagnosis, is not in the remit of the nurses or the health care team. Respecting Paul's autonomy and making decisions that are in his best interests necessitate a balance, weighing up whether telling his daughter of his terminal prognosis and diagnosis is going to benefit Paul or cause him further harm. The benefit of telling his daughter may cause greater harm and fracture the nurse–patient relationship. Here, the most just response may be that Paul's decision must be respected. Overriding this and telling his daughter would not be in his best interests.

Activity 6.10: Evidence-based practice

This scenario highlights some of the ethical dilemmas present. Staff may have differing views; however, what is important is that when discussing Henry's treatment with his family and relatives the information they provide is consistent. This will reduce the family's anxiety and promote clear communication. In addition the nurse needs to ensure that Henry's relatives are well informed and feel that they are involved in his care and treatment in a meaningful way. This will require the nurse, and other health care professionals, to demonstrate feelings of mutual trust and confidence between the patient and family.

Activity 6.11: Communication and decision-making

This scenario highlights some of the ethical dilemmas with research for participants in end of life and palliative care. The balance between the benefit and the risk must always be of paramount concern on the part of the researcher(s). Where capacity has an impact on participant consent then withdrawing of participation may be the right action to take, unless this can be achieved lawfully. No harm or inconvenience must come to the participant, even for the greater good of the findings from the research itself. This is a moral imperative.

Further reading

Casarett, D. (2005) Ethical considerations in end-of-life care and research. *Journal of Palliative Medicine*, 8 (S1): S148–S161.

This article discusses six ethical aspects of end of life care that clinicians and researchers should take into consideration when conducting palliative care research.

Chiarella, M. (2006) *Policy in EoLC: Education, Ethics, Practice and Research.* London: Quay.

This reference source provides a review on policy in end of life care.

Fry, S.T. and Johnstone, M.J. (2008) *Ethics in Nursing Practice: A Guide to Ethical Decision Making*, 3rd edn. Oxford: Blackwell.

This book will provide you with an in-depth understanding of the ethical, legal and professional issues that are key in supporting you to maintain professional standards.

Tschudin, V. (ed.) (2003) *Ethics in Nursing Beyond Boundaries*, 3rd edn. London: Butterworth Heinemann.

This text is a collection of contributions, from internationally recognised authors, on different approaches to ethics. These are written about and applied to nursing contexts.

Wheat, K. (2009) Applying ethical principles in healthcare practice. *British Journal of Nursing*, 18 (17): 1062–1063.

This article outlines general ethical principles that can be applied to all health care contexts.

Useful websites

www.hra.nhs.uk/news/dictionary/corec/

The Central Office for Research Ethics Committees' website contains useful information for health care professionals.

www.nmc-uk.org

This is the website for the Nursing and Midwifery Council. It contains relevant information about professional standards and guidance for practice.

www.rcn.org.uk

This is the website for the RCN, the largest professional union for nursing in the UK. Their website provides information on professional development and support.

www.scie.org.uk/consultancy/research

This website provides you with information about the Social Care Research Ethics Committee. It includes information about the research carried out and how to apply for research ethics review.

www.icn.ch

This website is the International Council for Nurses and provides you with the Code of Ethics for nurses.

www.legislation.gov.uk

This website provides access to all legislative instruments and serves as a main source to legal frameworks to guide lawful practice.

www.who.int/ethics/research/en/

This website provides current guidelines and standards for research ethics.

Chapter 7

Palliative and end of life care in a critical care setting

Hazel Luckhurst and Chris Clarke

NMC Standards for Pre-registration Nursing Education

This chapter will address the following competencies:

Domain 1: Professional values

1. All nurses must practise with confidence according to *The Code: Professional Standards of Practice and Behaviour for Nurses and Midwives* (NMC 2015), and within other recognised ethical and legal frameworks. They must be able to recognise and address ethical challenges relating to people's choices and decision-making about their care, and act within the law to help them and their families and carers find acceptable solutions.

Domain 2: Communication and interpersonal skills

3. All nurses must use the full range of communication methods, including verbal, non-verbal and written, to acquire, interpret and record their knowledge and understanding of people's needs. They must be aware of their own values and beliefs and the impact this may have on their communication with others. They must take account of the many different ways in which people communicate and how these may be influenced by ill health, disability and other factors, and be able to recognise and respond effectively when a person finds it hard to communicate.

Domain 3: Nursing practice and decision-making

4. All nurses must ascertain and respond to the physical, social and psychological needs of people, groups and communities. They must then plan, deliver and evaluate safe, competent, person-centred care in partnership with them, paying special attention to changing health needs during different life stages, including progressive illness and death, loss and bereavement.

4.2. Adult nurses must recognise and respond to the changing needs of adults, families and carers during terminal illness. They must be aware of how treatment goals and service users' choices may change at different stages of progressive illness, loss and bereavement.

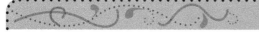

NMC Essential Skills Clusters

This chapter will address the following ESCs:

Cluster: Care, compassion and communication

2. People can trust the newly registered graduate nurse to engage in person-centred care empowering people to make choices about how their needs are met when they are unable to meet them for themselves.

Second progression point

6. Provides personalised care, or makes provision for those who are unable to maintain their own activities of living maintaining dignity at all times.

3. People can trust the newly registered graduate nurse to respect them as individuals and strive to help them preserve their dignity at all times.

Entry to the register

4. Acts professionally to ensure that personal judgements, prejudices, values, attitudes and beliefs do not compromise care.

Chapter aims

After reading this chapter you will be able to:

*   describe the three suggested phases relating to the management of a patient in critical care;
*   identify the challenges of introducing and caring for palliative care patients in a critical care environment;
*   reflect on the support required for the patient, family and critical care staff when delivering palliative and end of life care.

Introduction

I will never forget the day I walked into the critical care unit at the hospital to see my son. Simon had been in a road accident and the police brought us to the hospital ... What a shock. Even though the nurse had explained about Simon's bed area and the tubes before we walked in, I couldn't quite take it all in. As we got near to the bed my husband just collapsed and fell to the floor. We had to give him a few moments on the floor before sitting him up. He had fainted at the sight of Simon in the bed, all swollen, surrounded by machines and equipment.

(A mother's reflection on seeing her son for the first time following a road accident)

You may find the critical care environment alien and frightening; this is also true for families whose loved ones are being cared for in critical care. Simon's mother's words in the quote above recognise this. The focus is on the 'tubes' and 'machines', and the overt impact of this environment on Simon's parents is emphasised by his father's collapse.

Activity 7.1   *Reflection*

Take a few moments, either on your own or within a group, to reflect on what the intensive care environment means to you, both visually and in the sounds you may hear.

Brief answers to all activities are given at the end of the chapter, unless otherwise indicated. This activity is based on your own observations, so there is no outline answer given.

You may have included words like 'technical', 'equipment' or 'frightening' in your reflection in Activity 7.1, and possibly think that a critical care unit would be a very quiet healing environment. However, critical care units tend to be very busy and noisy and you should also consider that, as well as the general background noise, there is also considerable unexpected intermittent noises from medical alarms and from oxygen and suctioning.

All critically ill patients have cables and leads attaching them to monitoring equipment that displays their vital signs. The screens on the equipment display several coloured waveforms and are linked to specific haemodynamics of the patient, including the heart rhythm, arterial blood pressure and pulse oximetry. Patients receive intravenous infusions and may have several cannulae infusing fluids for hydration, as well as medication via syringe infusion pumps. As many of the patients are unable to eat for long periods of time, they are given liquid nutrients via a naso-gastric tube. Additional therapies may also be present at the bedside, such as a renal support machine and a ventilator supporting the patient's breathing.

Patients in a critical care setting are obviously critically ill, usually with a condition that is reversible, although not always. Sometimes there is the need to introduce the principles for palliative and end of life care discussed in Chapter 1. However, whatever the setting, be it home, hospital ward or critical care, you should look beyond the machines and equipment and afford the *patient, family* and *carers* the best possible care. You should also recognise that if you select critical care as a career choice it is important to know that around 20 per cent of patients may not survive their admission (Intensive Care Society 2011), and therefore end of life care is a substantial aspect of day-to-day care for the critical care nurse.

What is a critical care setting?

Within this chapter we will refer to the critical care unit as the intensive care unit (ICU), although in health care 'critical care' is carried out in many areas within a hospital, including the operating theatre or Emergency Department.

Level of care	Place of care
Level 0	Patients whose needs can be met through a normal ward setting
Level 1	Patients at risk of their condition deteriorating, or needing higher levels of care, whose need can be met with advice and support from the critical care team
Level 2	Patients requiring more detailed observation or intervention (single failing organ system) or postoperative care, and higher levels of care
Level 3	Patients requiring advanced respiratory support alone or basic respiratory support together with support of at least two organ systems. This level includes all complex patients requiring support for multiorgan failure

Table 7.1: Defined levels of care (DoH 2000)

The goal of critical care is ultimately to support and treat reversible causes of critical illness (Pattison 2011), maintaining life and relieving suffering (McLeod 2014). However, it has taken a considerable time to define what happens in ICUs around the UK because of the variation in patient criteria, reason for admission and speciality of some ICUs. To support ease of understanding across health care settings, a national review by the Department of Health took place in 2000. This review defined four levels of care throughout the hospital services (DH 2000) (Table 7.1).

Patients requiring level 2 and 3 support are usually nursed in an ICU. This is because they need potentially life-saving measures requiring staff with specialist skills and knowledge, in addition to the use of medical technology. As medicine and the speciality of critical care have advanced, subspecialties of intensive care have evolved. For example, a large university teaching hospital could have more than one ICU. The units may be named according to their speciality, for example, neurosciences critical care unit, cardiothoracic critical care unit, paediatric and trauma critical care unit.

Within the last decade the profile of end of life care within the ICU has been more evident in both UK and international policy and publications (DH 2008; Chapman 2009; Stayt 2009; Coombs et al. 2012). According to the Health and Social Care Information Centre (2016) in 2014–15 around 9 per cent of patients admitted to ICU died. For many health care professionals a patient's deterioration to the point of dying may be perceived as a sense of failure, however patients may die suddenly during efforts to provide curative treatment, or over an extended time, when collaborative decisions are required to move the focus of care towards comfort, quality of life and effective symptom management. The key role of the critical care nurse in end of life care though is to advocate for the patient, manage symptoms, and participate in educating the family, by encouraging and supporting family presence and the creation of positive memories (Arbour and Wiegand 2014).

Phases of care in critical care

In terms of planning and implementing holistic patient-centred care, nursing patients in an ICU is no different from other health care settings. However, there are some differences that should be recognised. First, medical technology and interventions actively support and can even replace the function of some organ systems during the severe stages of organ failure. Second, it is often not possible to involve patients in discussions about their care as they are seriously ill, at times unconscious and may be unable to communicate. Third, the serious illness may have developed rapidly, within minutes or hours, and finally, other services such as a hospice or palliative care teams may have had more time to plan end of life care with the patient and loved ones.

The discussion above and national statistics indicate that mortality in an ICU is high. This is why nurses, and other health care staff working in critical care, can be regularly providing end of life care. Using a framework could be helpful for you when considering the process of palliative care in critical care. One framework is described by Coombs et al. (2012), who discuss a specific trajectory involving three phases of care in critical care. Each phase will now be described using a supportive case scenario to illustrate what happens in each phase. Phase 0 is not discussed as it is technically not applicable to the intensive care environment.

Phase 1: hope of recovery

Patients are admitted to the critical care environment because there is *hope of recovery*. This hope of recovery is demonstrated in the example below.

> ### Case study: Phillip
>
> *Phillip was a 54-year-old business man, who was married with two teenage daughters. He awoke in the early hours of the morning with chest pain, and went downstairs to get a drink. His wife, Emma, heard a sudden crash and ran downstairs to find him collapsed on the floor. Phillip had had a heart attack and was no longer breathing. Having dialled 999 she was guided through the process of providing cardio-pulmonary resuscitation (CPR) over the telephone until the paramedics arrived to take over his care. Phillip was successfully resuscitated by the paramedics and, following intubation and ventilation to support his breathing, he was transferred to the hospital for further treatment prior to being admitted to the ICU.*

Activity 7.2   *Reflection*

- Consider the range of emotions Emma and other family members will be experiencing at the various stages of this scenario.
- What physical and psychological support will this family need when they arrive at the hospital and prior to being taken into ICU to see Phillip?

Looking at this example you may want to argue that this phase does not really require palliative care, as there is still hope for recovery. It is only if Phillip's condition deteriorates that he might move to phase 2, the transition phase.

Case study: Phillip

Twenty-four hours later both the ICU consultant and the cardiology consultant agreed that despite all best efforts, the damage to Phillip's heart and the deficit of oxygen to his brain was so extensive that further treatment would be considered futile.

Phase 2: the transition stage

This involves recognition that the treatment is not effective in the planned recovery of the patient as interventions have not resulted in an improvement of the patient's condition. There is a process of acknowledgement and a diagnosis that the person is dying. When a patient's condition is worsening health care professionals often review the care and treatment options for that patient. At times some forms of treatment become futile and it takes courage and knowledge to decide against futile treatment. The word futile may not be the easiest to understand, but when used in the caring environment it has a specific meaning. For example, if the multidisciplinary team you work with talks about the current treatment being futile, they mean that the treatment/intervention that the person is receiving is not having a positive effect (*Mosby's Medical Dictionary* 2009). Recognising the futility of treatment is the fundamental aspect of phase 2 in relation to the management of the patient (for further information on non-beneficence see Chapter 6).

In Phillip's case (phase 2) his organs were failing and therefore a decision to withdraw treatment would be made as part of the care plan. There are guidelines (Intensive Care Society 2003) which should be followed when this decision is made. They state that there should be agreement from two senior doctors, with one of the doctors being an intensive care consultant (Cohen et al. 2003). The guidelines also acknowledge that it is 'normal practice' for the opinions of the nursing and other medical team members to be considered. This shared decision-making process is supported by a survey carried out by McAree and Doherty in 2010.

Whilst maximum treatment therapies continue the focus moves to discussions with the nursing team and family members to reach a collaborative agreement to initiate the transition from cure to treatment withdrawal. However, the timelines of initiating end-of-life care in ICU can be difficult to manage and subsequent delays may challenge the quality of dying (Pattison et al. 2013). The delivery of care must move from replacing activities aimed towards the goal of curing with new processes orientated towards ensuring a comfortable death for the patient and supporting the family to come to terms with what is happening (Gallagher et al. 2015). When this decision is made, be careful what terminology is used. It is preferable to say 'withdrawing active therapy' rather than 'withdrawal of treatment', because whatever phase patients are in, they are still receiving treatment. Phillip, for example, will continue to receive analgesia and some support from the ventilator.

Activity 7.3   *Critical thinking*

Reflect on Phillip's case study.

- What possible feelings might you as the professional experience in this situation?
- What strategies could you put in place to address these and support yourself?

Activity 7.3 might have highlighted to you the emotional dilemma that nurses and other professionals working in a critical care setting face. Whilst it is the medical staff who have the authority to make a diagnosis of dying, it is essential to work collaboratively and gain consensus across the health care team in order to facilitate a patient and family-centric approach. The death of a patient is a devastating and life changing experience for many families, however it can be equally challenging for you as a nurse to make that transition from active treatment to palliation and end of life care. Conflict, though rare, may be related to medical uncertainty and disagreement between professional teams (Pattison et al. 2013), lack of collaborative decision-making (McLeod 2015) and the dissent of family members. Long-Sutehall et al. (2011) maintain that critical care nurses are often excluded from withdrawal of treatment decisions, however in contrast Gallagher et al. (2015) highlight that if experienced nurses feel certain that continued treatment is futile they may coax physicians to make decisions to withdraw or limit treatment by expressing their views.

Throughout the patient's stay, it is possible and most likely that you will have developed a rapport with the family and close friends of the patient, even over a short period of time. In ICU the nurse is constantly at the patient's bedside, placing you in the ideal position to tailor the key information given to relatives, to enable them to be actively involved in the decision-making, as well as helping to bring about acceptance of the situation, while having an awareness of their needs and feelings (Intensive Care Society 2003; Coombs et al. 2012). This can be an emotional time for you too though; it is important, therefore, that all health care professionals and nurses in particular have ways to self-care and debrief during or after each shift.

Phase 3: a controlled death

The term 'controlled death' could conjure up different meanings, including helping someone to die, which would be misconstruing what Coombs et al. (2012) and others had in mind. The phrase 'controlled death' should be viewed as allowing death to take place in a dignified way, through palliation to ease pain and suffering, recognising the suddenness of the death and the different meaning this has for people. It is necessary to emphasise here that Coombs et al. (2012) expand upon the term as a time of palliation, allowing nature to take its course, saying goodbye and returning the dead person to his or her family.

Case study: Phillip

Phillip arrived in the critical care unit four hours after his heart attack but despite 24 hours of aggressive treatment the extensive damage to his heart muscle meant that he would not recover. The critical care team discussed the situation with Phillip's family and end of life care was commenced. The priority was to care for Phillip, maintaining his dignity and comfort until his death.

Phillip's situation is classified here as phase 3. The length of time a patient spends in each of the three phases will vary depending upon the individual patient and condition. For example, you could be working alongside your mentor, nursing a patient in phase 1 for several weeks before the patient recovers or deteriorates and moves into phase 2. Some patients, like Phillip, may move from phase 1 through to phase 3 very quickly, in a matter of hours (Coombs et al. 2012). The point to make is how quickly conditions can change and therefore decision-making by intensive care staff needs to be equally prompt to reflect the changing dynamics.

Activity 7.4   *Critical thinking*

A seminal piece of research in 1979 by Molter identified that the three most important requirements of families whose relatives are in critical care are assurance, information and proximity. This identifies the family's need to feel cared for, informed and close to the patient.

As a nurse caring for Phillip and his family, how can you incorporate Molter's three requirements into your support for Emma and her sons?

In Activity 7.4 you might have identified areas like providing information to the family and allowing the family to visit at flexible times. These are all aspects of the care that is included once a patient is in phase 3 of the trajectory. The aim is to ensure comfort, peace and a dignified death. It is widely recognised that the majority of critically ill patients who are in phase 2 of the trajectory discussed above are unconscious (Curtis and Vincent 2010). However, the plan of care will be explained to patients, irrespective of their level of consciousness. It is believed that hearing is the last sense to go when patients become unconscious, so it is important that health care professionals assume patients can still hear and communicate with them accordingly. This may involve both verbal and non-verbal communication – touch when talking to them and verbal communication to inform them what you are doing.

Nursing the dying patient in critical care

The importance of the design of an ICU cannot be underestimated and should include planning for space and private rooms for a grieving family. However, the design of ICUs varies across the UK, where the number of beds in open spaces, the layout and the number of single rooms will all differ. These physical limitations can prove challenging in maintaining dignity and support for the relatives when providing palliative and end of life care. A large open-area bay may be occupied by several critically ill patients, with each 'bed space' separated only by curtains for screening and privacy. If there is an available single room the patient may be moved from an open area to a single room to enable a greater level of privacy. However, this is not always possible as single rooms are frequently occupied by patients requiring isolation due to infection. Recognising the need for privacy at this time should be considered; curtains and screens can only provide so much privacy. Thompson et al. (2012) recommend that places away from the ICU area should be made available so that a 'quiet space' is available for relatives. In most cases relatives can understand the physical limitations of the ICU, but staff need to reiterate this point to them as a way of acknowledging how difficult it might be for them not being close to the patient. This also enhances communication between staff and the relatives.

Removal of monitoring equipment

When active therapy is withdrawn the audible and visual alarm systems from the monitoring systems may be switched off to enable the focus of care to be on the patient and their family rather than on the machines. This might not always be the case; some critical care settings switch monitoring screens off and remove them from the bedside while others continue or reduce monitoring (McAree and Doherty 2010; Woodrow 2011). Removing equipment and machinery from the bedside seems to promote a peaceful and dignified setting for the patient and family. This action is congruent with Coombs et al.'s (2012) description of returning the person to the family, and it can present an almost tangible effect on the family becoming closer to the patient. In contrast to other health care settings, some patients may die within minutes or hours after active therapy is withdrawn. This can be influenced by factors such as the severity of organ failure and how dependent the patient was on supportive therapy. When the family are not at the bedside you may often see the nurse sitting with the patient and holding his or her hand (McCallum and McConigley 2013). This simple gesture, the use of therapeutic touch, supports the principle of ensuring a patient does not die alone.

Patients who are intubated and require ventilation continue to receive some respiratory support from a ventilator. However, the percentage of oxygen being administered may be reduced. It is rare for a patient to be extubated (McAree and Doherty 2010); the overall aim of maintaining ventilator support is to avoid distressing the patient and to reduce dyspnoea.

Communication and palliative care in critical care

Case study

Many of the patients admitted to ICU recover quickly; however, some patients remain critically ill for a significant period of time, which can have a lasting impact on their quality of life when they recover. For some patients though there can be a long period of uncertainty, where the patient's condition can quickly alter between appearing to recover before deteriorating again. For the family members this instability, and the fluctuation between phase 1 and phase 2 can be a very challenging time and they may experience feelings of stress, sadness and fatigue (Day et al. 2013). When the transition to phase 3 is eventually considered this may even be perceived as a relief. Having time to understand the severity of the patient's illness can help with understanding the complexities of the decision-making process.

Steve

Steve was an elective admission to the critical care unit following major surgery to repair an aortic aneurysm. Postoperatively Steve developed sepsis and remained critically ill for five weeks, requiring renal replacement therapy. The specific interventions to treat this sepsis and support his failing organ systems were not effective. Throughout the five weeks of Steve's stay in the ICU the staff had developed a rapport with his family. The family had had regular meetings with the staff since admission to discuss Steve's plan of care and recognised that his condition was worse.

Steve's wife (Diane)

I felt relief when the doctors and nurses talked to us about Steve. Going into the unit every day and seeing him there in the middle of all that technology trying to get him better ... Time went by and all the treatment was tried but sometimes you have to just accept it ... We talked through Steve's condition and the staff explained things. We felt the pressure was off us as the consultant described what was going to happen and also gave us some time to come to terms and make some plans. He had fought so hard but the sepsis was just too much ...

Like any patient, the patient with chronic critical illness has the right to make decisions about treatments that may be offered by the health care team. Ensuring and maintaining excellent communication between staff and relatives is crucial when caring for the dying patient in critical care. The overwhelming nature of the setting and the situation can mean that conversations with relatives are forgotten or information is misunderstood. Documentation of meetings needs to be clear and consistent, and should include the date and time of the meeting, names of staff and family present, the issues discussed and comments made by the family and staff. To improve communication between members of the health care team and with the relatives it is good practice for all meetings to include both a member of the nursing team and one of the doctors involved in the care of the patient. This ensures that members of the team are aware of what has been said to the family, can offer consistent support and can promote continuity of care between different shifts, including on-call staff.

Effective and supportive communication can support the family to ask questions and clarify any concerns they have. In addition the length of stay for the patient in critical care often influences the amount of information given and the development of rapport between staff and the patient's family and close friends. It is clearly acknowledged that you, as the nurse, are best placed to know the views of the relatives (Coombs and Long 2008; Coombs et al. 2012). The nurse caring for the dying patient will ascertain and document important information about the family and the patient to assist the plan of care. The information will include spiritual care and detail relating to family members wishing to be present at the bedside when death occurs.

Activity 7.5   *Evidence-based practice and research*

During your next practice placement take the time to visit the ICU in the hospital where you are working. Discuss with staff how palliative care is practised and what documentation is used to support palliative and end of life care in their setting.

As this activity is based on your own observations, there is no outline answer at the end of this chapter.

Whichever approach you find in Activity 7.5, the key aim must be for clear, precise communication with all involved and for all health care professionals to be familiar with the process. Currently there is variation in the documentation used and how the stages of end of life care are managed. Some critical care units have developed specific well-established NHS trust protocols or tools. Some follow broad principles of the national strategy (DH 2008). A new approach to caring for dying people based on the needs and wishes of the person and those close to them is the One Chance to Get it Right report, written by the Leadership Alliance for the Care of the Dying Patient (LACDP 2014), to encourage a more individualised care pathway, reflecting openness, transparency and candour, that further enhances communication and involvement in decision-making.

The report highlights five priorities of care:

1. The possibility that a person may die within the next few days or hours is recognised and communicated clearly, decisions made and actions taken in accordance with the person's needs and wishes, and these are regularly reviewed and decisions revised accordingly.
2. Sensitive communication takes place between staff and the person who is dying and those identified as important to them.
3. The dying person and those identified as important to them are involved in decisions about treatment and care to the extent that the dying person wants.
4. The needs of families and others identified as important to the dying person are actively explored, respected and met as far as possible.
5. An individual plan of care, which includes food and drink, symptom control and psychological, social and spiritual support, is agreed, coordinated and delivered with compassion.

In addition to this is the relatively new concept directed at facilitating the transfer of palliative care patients from the ICU back to their home environment to die (Lusardi et al. 2011; Coombs et al. 2015). Whilst this may be a good idea in principle, it is also a complex and time-dependent process involving rapid discharge and enhanced communication between health care agencies across both primary and secondary care settings (Coombs et al. 2015).

Involving the family in the care

Family members and friends whose relatives are receiving palliative and end of life care in an ICU setting often experience feelings of helplessness. They may want to be more actively involved in some of the practical aspects of the patient's care. The family may have already been involved in care during phase 1 (recovery) and phase 2 (transition) of active therapy. Family members can be involved in activities like assisting in administering mouth care, shaving and hair care. Support from you, by providing reassurance and expertise, will increase the relatives' confidence in carrying out these activities. As well as more practical activities, family members may also like to play music and should be encouraged to talk to the patient. If family members are unsure whether the dying person can hear them or not, always assume that the patient can hear. You will play an important role here in 'normalising' verbal communication with the patient, encouraging the family to talk naturally to the patient. Initially relatives may feel embarrassed and some members may be afraid to talk to the patient. By supporting relatives to talk to the patient you can assist the family to feel a 'connection' with him or her. Some family members may give simple updates of what is happening day to day in their community and others recognise it to be a time of saying goodbye and reminiscing about their time together. You should be sensitive to this need for privacy and take the time to physically 'stand back' from the bedside (Coombs et al. 2012).

Caring for yourself

The nurse-to-patient ratio of 1:1 or 1:2 in patient care in critical care reinforces the philosophy of holistic, patient-centred care. However, mortality rates are high, showing that palliative and end of life care can be a regular aspect of critical care nursing (Adam and Osborne 2005; Intensive Care National Audit and Research Centre 2010; Pattison et al. 2013).

Activity 7.6   *Reflection*

Reflect back on your answers to Activities 7.1 and 7.2 and answer the following questions:

- Did you consider that providing palliative and end of life care would feature regularly in a critical care setting? Why was that?
- Has your original view of critical care changed? If so, how?

As this activity is based on your own observations, there is no outline answer at the end of this chapter.

In your answer to Activity 7.6 you may have recognised the role that palliative and end of life care have in critical care and the impact of this on you. Doing this will encourage you to develop your knowledge and skills in this area. The other chapters in this book address many essential aspects of palliative and end of life care that you can use to support your care in an ICU setting.

The most challenging phase for you, and other nurses in critical care might be phase 2. When the decision to withdraw active treatment is made it is important that staff have confidence that everything was done for the patient and there is agreement in the decision making (McAree and Doherty 2010). You may not necessarily feel comfortable with the decision that has been made; however, you need to have confidence that the decision was the right one and was in the best interest of the patient. This may result in some tension between members of the health care team. This is often the case if the nurse feels that the decision-making process was delayed and therapy prolonged (Walker and Read 2010; Coombs et al. 2012). It should be recognised that decisions cannot always be made quickly. Some patients may be cared for by several clinical speciality teams and a consensus needs to be reached by all these teams. The decision to withdraw active treatment is not an easy one to make; positive, open interdisciplinary team work can support staff to understand and accept the rationale for the decision. Due to the nurse's very visible role at the bedside, McCallum and McConigley (2013) describe the nurse as the protector of the patient, with the aim of promoting a peaceful, dignified death in what can be a noisy environment.

A key aspect in terms of your personal well-being and performance and in staff retention is to have a supportive positive team ethos. It is widely recognised that critical care nurses require ongoing education and clinical supervision to address end of life care (Stayt 2009; Walker and Read 2010; Shannon et al. 2011; Woodrow 2011). This can be done formally through ongoing staff development and clinical supervision. Additionally, having time to debrief, as a team, is important; this can be done informally or in a more structured manner. Having the time to reflect on the care provided, the decisions made and how palliative and end of life care was managed is crucial for the wellbeing of staff and the continuity of care for future patients. You and your colleagues will respond in different ways to the death of a patient. Scholes (2006) recalls a situation where a doctor sat distressed, head in hands, during the end of life care of a patient. The impact on the doctor was one of dismay and a feeling of failure in not facilitating recovery. Rather than reflect on 'watching them die' the nurses and the team can be 'with' the dying person, ensuring comfort and peace.

Organ donation

Good end of life care planning enables patients to die with dignity, but will inevitably involve some difficult and sensitive decisions being made. In accordance with guidelines published by NICE (2016), organ donation should be considered as a usual part of end-of-life care planning and the doctors may choose to explore with family members whether the patient had expressed any views about organ donation.

One person can save or transform up to nine lives through organ donation. However, according to statistics from NHS Blood and Transplant (NHSBT), the UK still has one of the lowest rates of consent in Europe (NHSBT 2016), and consent from potential organ donors in ICUs has been recognised as a barrier to maximising the organ supply since transplantation became an available procedure (Goldberg et al. 2014). Sometimes this is because even though you have signed the Organ Donor Register, you may not have discussed this with your family and therefore they are not aware of your wishes. Having these conversations is important; it is vital your family know as they will be asked for consent. Indeed Nazarko (2016) maintains that even when a person has signed up to be a donor, around five per cent of families decline donation even when the donor has registered his or her wishes to donate. In the past five years, more than 500 families have declined to honour the wishes of donors and an estimated 1200 people missed out on a transplant that could potentially have saved their life (NHSBT 2016).

In an attempt to address the poor consent rates, the organ donation service was redesigned in 2008 and specialist nurses in organ donation (SN-ODs) were embedded into hospital trusts, supported in practice by a locally appointed clinical lead in organ donation (CL-OD). NICE guidelines (2016) state that a SN-OD should be involved in the planning and discussion of organ donation with the donor or their family, and early identification and referral helps to ensure this occurs. More recently NHSBT have introduced a new role, that of the SN-OD specialist requester, who specialises in family approach and gaining consent, to ensure families are given the best possible support when asked to consider donation on behalf of a loved one (NHSBT 2016).

Almost anyone dying in hospital is a potential organ or tissue donor and more people than ever before across the UK donated their organs after their deaths last year. In 2015/16, 1364 people became organ donors when they died and their donations resulted in 3519 transplants taking place (NHSBT 2016). In most countries death is defined by reference either to irreversible cessation of the circulatory system (asystole) or irreversible cessation of brain function (brain death) (Bendorf et al. 2013). Organ donation can occur in two different ways. When organs are procured from a patient in whom all brain function has ceased but a normal heart beat continues, it is referred to as donation after brain death (DBD). This may occur in patients who have had a catastrophic head injury, either from a medical or traumatic cause. Organ procurement after cessation of cardiac activity and cardiorespiratory function is referred to as donation after circulatory death (DCD). There are two types of DCD: controlled and uncontrolled. Controlled DCD refers to the retrieval of organs from a patient following planned withdrawal of life-sustaining treatments, as in the case of both Phillip and Steve discussed above. Uncontrolled DCD refers to the retrieval of organs from a patient who has had an unexpected cardiac arrest and from which the patient cannot or should not be resuscitated (NHSBT 2016).

Activity 7.7 — Reflection

More than 500 families in the UK have said no to organ donation taking place since 1 April 2010 despite knowing or being informed their relative was on the NHS Organ Donor Register and wanted to donate, and half the adults in England have never talked to anyone about their wishes (NHSBT 2016). In a recent UK study of 667 *continued ...* •

student nurses it was found that nearly half of the student cohort had registered as organ donors and that a further third would be willing to consider donation (McGlade et al. 2014). Given the fundamental role that nurses play in the organ donation process, consider the following:

1. Have you registered as an organ donor? Whether you agree with organ donation or not, have you shared your decision with other members of your family?
2. Do you know if any of your family and friends have registered? If not, consider having that conversation with them.
3. Visit the NHSBT website to find out more information: **www.organdonation.nhs.uk**.

As this activity is based on your own observations, there is no outline answer at the end of this chapter.

In Activity 7.7 you may have either asked yourself, or family members, difficult questions. If you are going to support families of patients who are dying to consider organ donation then it is important that you understand your own thoughts and feelings about this. To further develop your knowledge and understanding of organ donation during your next placement take the time to visit the ICU to find out how embedded the SN-OD role is.

Chapter summary

This chapter has provided an overview of the role that palliative and end of life care has in a critical care setting. The focus of ICU is primarily on maintaining life, with complex decisions being made to minimise suffering. For patients, and their families, being admitted to ICU initiates a sense of hope; however, the trajectory of the patient's journey can be very challenging and the transition from cure to end of life care may become the reality. The three phases of care have been discussed and applied to case studies; the challenge presented by phase 2 has been recognised and explored in relation to providing palliative and end of life care. Strategies to support families have been outlined, including promoting communication and family involvement in the care of the patient. It is always important in any care you give to know yourself (self-awareness). Being aware of your feelings and values, and how you respond, will impact on the care that you provide for your patients. Some patients' values and beliefs may not reflect your own, but you may have to accept these as a professional caring for your patients. Establishing a collaborative approach to end of life care is important in promoting family understanding of the situation, to ensure timely decisions are made without prolonging suffering. Where organ donation is a consideration, discussions should be led by the SN-OD or SN-OD specialist requester, who will have the necessary knowledge and skills to support the process and provide donor family care in accordance with best practice.

Activities: brief outline answers

Activity 7.2: Reflection

Emma will be experiencing a deep sense of shock in the events leading up to Phillip being admitted to the ICU but equally a sense of hope that he had been successfully resuscitated and was alive. The ICU environment can be anxiety provoking and emotionally distressing for all family members, particularly for younger children as visiting may be restricted. For Emma the stress of having to resuscitate her husband may lead to feelings of fear for how she will cope with the immediate external demands such as household and financial responsibilities and managing the needs of her family. Over time balancing the wish to be with her husband with the daily demands of family responsibilities can lead to family members becoming unwell themselves because of minimal sleep and lack of suitable food to eat and drink. Depression and post traumatic stress symptoms are common among ICU relatives.

Family members will need to be supported in basic physical needs as well as emotionally. You can help them by explaining what happens in the daily ICU routine and who people are as well as letting them know where the toilet is, where they can get something to eat and drink, visiting times and the direct line number for the ICU. Most ICUs will have written information for relatives detailing all this for them to refer back to, which is also a good resource for you to consider.

Activity 7.3: Critical thinking

You might have identified feelings of sadness, frustration and helplessness that there was no further treatment that could be provided for Phillip. Recognising this and taking positive steps to address this is key to maintaining your wellbeing and promoting professional development. It may be helpful to express your feelings to your mentor or the qualified staff you are working alongside. Many nurses will automatically pick up your cues as to how you are feeling, and it can also help to talk to your peers about the challenges you face. Remember staff, just as much as families, need time to process their emotions.

It may be possible (although rare) that you feel that Phillip would be at peace and not suffering anymore. You might have thought death was most appropriate given Phillip's deteriorating condition. In that case you would still need to 'listen' to yourself and how you are feeling at the time. It is always important to care for yourself in both good and bad outcomes to care.

Activity 7.4: Critical thinking

Assurance – providing reassurance to Phillip's family, being realistic, not too pessimistic or unrealistically optimistic about the situation. Giving Phillip's family time to ask any questions, talk about their situation and ask them what concerns them.

Information – providing appropriate information to Phillip's family, how much information they want: some people might want to know everything, whereas others might only want to know a little at a time. Ensuring they understand the information that is being provided.

Proximity – explaining the equipment to Phillip's family, allowing them to sit by him and to be physically close to him. Letting Phillip's family know that they can touch and talk to Phillip is also important in allowing his family to connect with him.

Further reading

Bloomer, M., Morphet, J., O'Conner, M., Lee, S. and Griffiths, D. (2013) Nursing care of the family before and after a death in the ICU: an exploratory pilot study. *Australian Critical Care*, 26 (1): 23–28.

The focus of this article explores how nurses working in ICU care for families and the strategies they use to ensure person-centred family care.

Lusardi, P., Jodka, P., Stambovsky, M., Stadnicki, B., Babb, B., Plouffe, D., Doubleday, N., Pizlak, Z., Walles, K. and Montonye, M. (2011) The going home initiative: getting critical care patients home with hospice. *Critical Care Nurse*, 31 (5): 46–57.

This article discusses how an ICU palliative care team developed guidelines to support getting patients home from ICU with hospice care.

Stayt, L.C. (2009) Death, empathy and self-preservation: the emotional labour of caring for families of the critically ill in adult intensive care. *Journal of Clinical Nursing*, 18: 1267–1275.

A study of the impact on nurses supporting patients and their families in critical care and subsequent recommendations.

Useful websites

www.baccn.org.uk

The British Association of Critical Care Nurses promotes the art and science of critical care nursing. The association works in collaboration in professional development and policy making.

www.gmc-uk.org/guidance/ethical_guidance/end_of_life_care.asp

This site provides information on *Treatment and Care Towards End of Life: Good Practice in Decision Making* (2010) and includes information on withdrawing treatment.

www.ics.ac.uk/ics

This is the homepage for the Intensive Care Society. This body represents intensive care professionals and promotes the delivery of quality care for patients in critical care settings. Their guidelines and standards section has information on bereavement in critical care and other aspects of palliative and end of life care.

www.organdonation.nhs.uk

This is the homepage for the UK organ donation website where you will find more information about organ donation, including some real life stories.

Chapter 8
Legal aspects of palliative and end of life care

Helen Taylor

NMC Standards for Pre-registration Nursing Education

This chapter will address the following competencies:

Domain 1: Professional values

1. All nurses must practise according to *The Code: Professional Standards of Practice and Behaviour for Nurses and Midwives* (NMC 2015), and within other recognised ethical and legal frameworks. They must be able to recognise and address ethical challenges relating to people's choices and decision-making about their care, and act within the law to help them and their families and carers find acceptable solutions.

2. All nurses must practise in a holistic, non-judgemental, caring and sensitive manner that avoids assumptions; supports social inclusion; recognises and respects individual choice; and acknowledges diversity. Where necessary, they must challenge inequality, discrimination and exclusion from care.

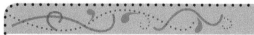

NMC Essential Skills Clusters

This chapter will address the following ESCs:

Cluster: Organisational aspects of care

11. People can trust the newly registered graduate nurse to safeguard children and adults from vulnerable situations and support and protect them from harm.

First progression point

1. Acts within legal frameworks and local policies in relation to safeguarding adults and children who are in vulnerable situations.

By the second progression point

4. Documents concerns and information about people who are in vulnerable situations.

Entry to the register

9. Supports people in asserting their human rights.

10. Challenges practices which do not safeguard those in need of support and protection.

Chapter aims

After reading this chapter you will be able to:

- explore the legal basis of a nurse's obligation to provide patient care;
- appreciate the importance of patient autonomy;
- explain the law in relation to consent and refusal to consent;
- reflect on legal issues relating to the sanctity of life;
- evaluate and define circumstances where treatment may lawfully be withdrawn or withheld.

Introduction

Case study: Amy

Amy is 42 years old, and is married to Adam with two pre-school-aged children. She is a physiotherapist and has always been fit and active. She has been a marathon runner, and competed regularly in tri-athlons. Three years ago she was diagnosed with motor neurone disease (MND), which has progressed rapidly. She is no longer able to work or participate in the activities that she used to enjoy. She is cared for at home by Adam, who has given up his job as an accountant. Since her diagnosis, Amy has focused on the target of living long enough to see her son and daughter start school.

Amy is now doubly incontinent, and has severely impaired mobility. She has an in-dwelling urinary catheter, and has been admitted to your ward with a urinary tract infection. She is pyrexial and in considerable discomfort. This is the fourth time she has been admitted for treatment of an infection in recent months. Shortly before her intravenous infusion of antibiotics is due to commence, Amy calls one of the nurses over and says that she no longer wants to have this treatment. She insists she knows she is going to die anyway, and she would rather it is now. She knows that with treatment she is likely to recover from the infection, but go on to experience the inevitably prolonged, difficult and undignified end to her life that is likely to result from her neurological condition. She tells the nurse that, although she is devastated at the prospect of not seeing her children grow up, she would rather she and her family were spared what she considers to be a 'horrific and torturous' death. Amy is adamant that she wants the health professionals 'just to let her go' and not treat the infection.

Activity 8.1	*Reflection*

Now, imagine you are the nurse Amy has summoned to her bedside for this conversation. Think about how you might respond to what she is saying.

Undertaking the reflection in Activity 8.1 will provide you with a baseline in relation to your knowledge and confidence regarding legal aspects of palliative care. This chapter will support you to develop your knowledge and confidence relating to legal issues in palliative and end of life care. No consideration of end of life care would be complete without exploring the impact of law on the delivery of care, for example issues relating to consent to treatment and an individual's capacity to consent. However, whereas consent is a matter to be considered for all patients, regardless of their health status and general condition, there are some legal issues that relate only to those approaching the end of their lives, such as the withholding of life-sustaining treatment.

As a health care professional, accepting that your patient is dying may be difficult. This may be particularly challenging if you have got to know the patient and their family well, but recognising that a life is coming to an end is likely to be upsetting, even if it does relieve the patient from great pain and other distressing symptoms (Taylor 2015). In addition to managing the sadness of a life ending, you may also feel challenged by some of the decisions made when caring for someone in the final stages of life, and be uncomfortable with the transition from active to palliative care. You would not be alone in experiencing concerns about some elements of end of life care, such as withdrawing clinically assisted nutrition and hydration (CANH), and you may be aware of the professional, public and media focus on the now obsolete Liverpool Care Pathway (LCP).

This increased attention to often very difficult decisions associated with end of life care culminated in an independent review of the LCP which recommended that generic protocols for the care of the dying be replaced with individualised plans of care, supported by practice guidelines (Independent Review of the Liverpool Care Pathway 2013). The 'One Chance to Get it Right' Agenda (Leadership Alliance for the Care of Dying People 2014) replaced the LCP from summer 2014, and focuses on individualised care that *reflect[s] the needs and preferences of the dying person and those who are important to them* rather than *generic protocols* (Leadership Alliance for the Care of Dying People 2014: 7). The agenda rests on five priorities for the fulfilment of compassionate care, including clear and sensitive communication, and the involvement of the patient and those important to them in the decisions underpinning an individualised plan of care.

Despite all this, some health care professionals will continue to experience a sense of discomfort when attempts at curative treatments and even basic life support end. It is counterintuitive: from the moment you embarked on your career, the instinct is to act to preserve life. How can it be that on the one hand it may be permissible, and entirely appropriate, to discontinue intravenous infusion of fluids, whereas on the other it is unlawful to administer an intramuscular injection of diamorphine with the intention of terminating someone's life, regardless of how much pain that person is in?

This chapter will give you the opportunity to understand how the law applies in a variety of end of life care scenarios.

Obligation to treat

Before going on to consider the law as it relates specifically to end of life care, it is important to understand some fundamental legal issues. For example, there are a number of categories of law, but the two that this chapter will focus on are criminal and civil law. These two areas of law have some significant differences. The aim of criminal law is to impose state requirements for the conduct of its citizens in order to maintain order and enable public protection, whilst the aim of civil law is to enforce obligations (e.g., contract, trespass and negligence) between individuals and/or organisations. A breach of the criminal law may result in an action being brought by the state, and if a prosecution is successful, punishments such as imprisonment, fines, community orders, rehabilitation orders, and many more, may be imposed. Conversely, an action for breach of civil law can be brought by any individual or organisation affected by the breach, and if successful may result in compensation being awarded for any loss resulting from this breach (Slapper and Kelly 2015).

Negligence (civil law)

The primary focus of this chapter will be on civil law – the obligations that exist between an individual (or organisation) and other individuals (or organisations). These legal responsibilities may arise in a number of ways. For example, if you enter into a contract with a decorator to paint the front of your house for £600, you will have a legal obligation to pay them £600 when the work is completed. In turn, the decorator will be required to complete the work as specified in the contract. Similarly, if you buy an item from an online store, the store has an obligation to ensure the item you receive is as described. In these two examples the obligations arise from a clearly recognisable and formal contract, with much of the detail of each party's obligations specified either verbally or in writing. Sometimes, however, civil law obligations do not come from any form of written or verbal contract, but arise from a particular situation rather than any formally recognised relationship (Halsbury's Laws of England 2010). This area of civil law is known as *tort*, and one example is negligence, as explained by Lord Aitkin in *Donoghue* v *Stevenson* ([1932]: 580):

> *You must take reasonable care to avoid acts or omissions which you can reasonably foresee would be likely to injure your neighbour. Who then, in law, is my neighbour? The answer seems to be – persons who are so closely and directly affected by my act that I ought reasonably to have them in contemplation as being so affected when I am directing my mind to the acts or omissions which are called into question.*

By recognising the possibility that an individual (you may not know who the person is) or a general group of people could be affected by your actions or failure to act, you have established a duty of care to these people – your 'neighbours' in law. Your response will be judged against the standard of the 'reasonable person' – a legal test which considers 'is this what a reasonable person either would or would not have done?' (*Blyth* v *The Company of Proprietors of the Birmingham Waterworks* [1856]). This means that you have a legal responsibility to ensure that your acts, or omissions, do not cause harm to anyone you could reasonably anticipate being affected by your actions, or failure to act, in a particular situation.

A useful way of summarising the application of the general law of negligence is to ask yourself:

1. Does a duty of care exist?
2. Has it been breached (either by doing something or failing to do something that a reasonable person would either have done or not done)?
3. Has harm been suffered?
4. Is this harm of a type that is reasonably foreseeable?

If you answer yes to each of these questions, you may be liable in negligence.

Scenario

As you are sitting at Amy's bedside, you are called over by another patient who urgently needs a vomit bowl. As you stand up, you accidentally bump into another patient's bedside table and tip over a plastic beaker of water. The spillage of water very small. You deliberate for a moment but decide that you will come back later to mop up the spillage.

Although you intend to return and clean up the water later, by leaving it, there is a risk that colleagues, patients or visitors to the ward might slip on the spillage and injure themselves. By creating a potentially dangerous situation (spilling the water) you have established a duty of care to people likely to be affected by this – other individuals using the corridor. Most reasonable people would ensure that the water was mopped up in order to remove the hazard. If you did not do that, you breached your duty of care to other people passing through the ward. If someone were to slip and sustain an injury (which could reasonably be foreseen as the result of slipping on a hard floor), then you might be liable in negligence.

Activity 8.2   *Decision-making*

Apply the test of negligence in these situations. On the evidence provided, do you think there may be liability in negligence?

1. You are sitting in the hospital library, and are engrossed in this book. You eat a banana while you read, and are so eager to finish this chapter that you drop the banana skin onto the floor next to you. Hanna is hurrying out of the library as she is running late

continued …

for the start of her shift, and does not see the banana skin on the floor. She slips on it and unfortunately fractures her wrist. As a result she has to defer her final surgical examinations, and misses out on a much anticipated promotion. In her spare time Hanna enjoys rowing, but is not able to participate in an important event for which she has spent the past four months training.

2. You are upset by the incident in the library, and decide to go for a relaxing walk in the countryside. You cross a field full of pregnant sheep, and walk through a gateway on to a winding lane. You do not close the gate behind you, and the sheep escape into the lane. A group of cyclists riding down the lane are met by a large flock of sheep as they round a bend. All three of them are unable to stop their bikes safely and fall, sustaining injuries ranging from cuts and brusies to a fractured collar bone. Their bikes are damaged. The sheep become very distressed, and a number later miscarry their lambs. An on-coming car also suffers damage when the driver (unharmed, but shaken) drives into a tree as he swerves to avoid the sheep.

An outline answer is given at the end of this chapter.

Clinical negligence

The previous examples of negligence come from daily life, but for you, as a health care professional, special rules apply. Health care professionals have a civil law duty to deliver care with reasonable competence and skill, as measured against the standards of other *reasonably competent [practitioners] at the time* (*Bolam* v *Friern Hospital Management Committee* [1957]: 121) (to be referred to as *Bolam* [1957]). Originally the judgement in *Bolam* [1957] referred explicitly to doctors and the medical profession, but since then it has been applied more broadly to all health care professionals (Halsbury's Laws of England 2011), and there is a wide body of case law which explores and defines this duty. For example, the case of *Cassidy* v *Ministry of Health* ([1951] p360), where Lord Denning made clear his opinion on the responsibilities of health care providers:

> [A]uthorities who run a hospital, be they local authorities, government boards, or any other corporation, are in law under the self-same duty as the humblest doctor; whenever they accept a patient for treatment, they must use reasonable care and skill to cure him of his ailment. The hospital authorities cannot, of course, do it by themselves: they have no ears to listen through the stethoscope, and no hands to hold the surgeon's knife. They must do it by the staff which they employ; and if their staff are negligent in giving the treatment, they are just as liable for that negligence as is anyone else who employs others to do his duties for him. What possible difference in law, I ask, can there be between hospital authorities who accept a patient for treatment, and railway or shipping authorities who accept a passenger for carriage? None whatever. Once they undertake the task, they come under a duty to use care in the doing of it, and that is so whether they do it for reward or not.

So, unlike general negligence, the parameters of clinical negligence are more clearly defined. For example, in a therapeutic relationship (unlike general negligence) there is unlikely to be much debate about the existence of a duty of care between you and your patient. Also, the standard of care will likely be higher. The test will not be the standard exercised by the 'reasonable person', but instead you will be judged against other nurses with the same education, training and skills.

Quite how this might be determined is a question that has been explored and debated at great length. The general position in law is still provided by a case that was decided more than 50 years ago in *Bolam* ([1957]: 122), where McNair J stated that *a doctor is not guilty of negligence if he has acted in accordance with a practice accepted as proper by a responsible body of medical men skilled in that particular art.*

Over the intervening years this test, now widely known as the 'Bolam test', has been subject to further refinement and clarification. In essence this means that the standard of care can now be more generally applied to all health care professionals, including nurses, and measured against what is regarded as reasonable and logical (*Bolitho* v *City and Hackney H.A.* [1997]) at the time the act or omission in question took place.

At this point it is worth mentioning that those working for organisations which sit outside the National Health Service – e.g., private hospitals and care agencies – may also be subject to leg-islation which regulates the provision of purchased services, such as the Consumer Rights Act (2015). However, regardless of the source of the law, there is an expectation that nurses will pro-vide care of a reasonable standard. This is in addition to the ethical and professional imperatives considered in Chapter 6 that will ensure that patients receive end of life care that is not only evidence-based, person-centred and of good quality. Activity 8.3 will prompt you to apply your problem-solving skills to your knowledge of legal issues.

Activity 8.3   *Critical thinking*

Read again the preceding paragraphs and think carefully about patients reaching the end of their life. Consider the words of Lord Denning, and make a note of any questions that come to your mind in response to his statement.

At the end of the chapter you should return to your list of questions and see how many remain unanswered. As a critical health care professional, your next task is to undertake further reading and investigation to answer those outstanding questions. The further read-ing at the end of the chapter is a good starting point.

As this activity is based on your own observations, there is no outline answer at the end of this chapter.

Consent in palliative and end of life care

Having read the previous section you will have noticed that the emphasis is very much on the role and responsibilities of both the health care provider (such as the hospital or hospice) and individual nurses and other health care professionals. One very important member of the care relationship has yet to be considered, and that of course is the patient. Talking about the imperative to deliver good-quality care completely disregards any recognition of patients' rights to involvement in decisions about their care. Although health care providers and professionals have a civil law obligation to make an offer of care, patients are generally under no legal obligation to accept that offer.

'Consent' is a word used widely in health care; voluntary provision of valid and informed consent is generally recognised as a necessary part of treatment. But why is consent so important?

Activity 8.4 — *Reflection*

Let us return now to Amy, the patient with motor neurone disease we met at the beginning of this chapter.

You know that although Amy is now refusing antibiotic treatment, she has accepted this on a least three occasions in the past – which gives us an opportunity to consider the issue of consent in practice. So, Amy was also diagnosed with a urinary tract infection on her previous admission. She had a temperature of 38.2°C and was experiencing significant discomfort. Once she had received all relevant test results, her doctor – Raschid – visited her to explain the diagnosis and available options. Amy asked if she could have oral antibiotics as she had sometimes experienced discomfort from having an intravenous cannula. Raschid explained that oral antibiotics were unlikely to be effective for such a serious infection, and would take too long to act. He considered that intravenous antibiotics was the preferred option: they would be faster acting and help reduce the possibility of further harm. Amy asked what the implications of not treating the infection would be, and Raschid explained these in detail. He went on to discuss the potential implications of intravenous therapy, and side-effects of the antibiotic. Amy told him that, as a physiotherapist herself, she understood what he had told her, and she consented both to the insertion of a cannula into her vein, and the administration of the antibiotics.

So, on this occasion Amy gave her consent to both the administration of intraveneous antibiotics and the route of administration. The information she gave when asking about the route of administration would have indicated that she understood what she was consenting to, and it was therefore appropriate for consent to be given orally. Raschid would need to make a record of this discussion however. The situation would be different if, for example, Raschid was proposing that Amy undergo a more significant surgical intervention – in which case it would be advisable for him to ask her to sign a record of the information sharing process as written evidence of consent. (The BMA has a useful toolkit on obtaining and evidencing patient consent – see the further reading section.) Consider too the very different circumstances described previously, when Amy stated she did not wish to receive intravenous antibiotics. Any treatment administered in those circumstances would be unlawful as Amy has decision-making capacity (MCA 2005). Although she has been fully informed about the risks and benefits, she has refused her consent (see the section on 'refusal of consent' below).

Now, think about some of the situations where you have witnessed a patient giving consent and reflect on the following:

- What was the patient consenting to? Did the patient know? Can you be sure of that? How?
- Did you know what the patient was consenting to? Did you need to know?
- How did the patient communicate consent? Was it always in the same way?
- Is it important that consent is given in the same way? Why?
- Were there any situations where treatment was given without the patient being asked for consent? Why? What did you think about that? Why?

As this activity is based on your own observations, there is no outline answer at the end of this chapter.

Activity 8.4 allowed you to reflect on the importance of consent and what it means to the therapeutic relationship between you and your patients. The importance of a patient giving voluntary, informed consent before receiving any form of treatment or therapeutic intervention is underpinned by the ethical and legal principle of self-determination (see Chapter 6). Lord Goff stated: *The fundamental principle, plain and incontestable, is that every person's body is inviolate* (*Collins* v *Wilcock* [1984]: 378). This means we all have the right to decide who touches our body, and any touching without our consent is generally unlawful. This principle is so important that unusually, touching without consent (referred to in law as 'battery') may constitute a breach of both criminal and civil law. Even putting someone in fear of non-consensual touching is unlawful, and is known as an 'assault' (Halsbury's Laws of England 2015).

This terminology can be confusing, but because 'assault' is usually synonymous with 'battery', the general tendency is to adopt the term 'assault' for both offences (*Fagan* v *Metropolitan Police Commissioner* [1968]), you will often hear the offence referred to as 'common assault'. Although both crimes originated from the common law, they are now enshrined in section 39 of the Criminal Justice Act 1988 and constitute summary offences.

Consent therefore serves as a legal defence – a legal 'safety blanket' that makes lawful what would otherwise be unlawful. There are some other defences to assault and battery, such as self-defence; prevention of crime; protection of property and the lawful chastisement of a child. Without valid consent, any touching of a patient's body will therefore be unlawful. Other than in some exceptional circumstances (which will be detailed below) consent is required before any treatment or therapeutic intervention can lawfully take place.

What is valid consent?

As identified in Activity 8.4 where you considered the circumstances of Amy's care, and your own reflections on situations you have encountered in practice, consent will only be valid if it has been freely given by a fully informed person who has the capacity to make that decision. Patients must be told both the risks and the benefits associated with the proposed treatment or intervention (*Montgomery* v *Lanarkshire Health Board* [2015]; *Chester* v *Afshar* [2004]), be able to evaluate that information and then communicate their decision.

The rules regarding decision-making capacity differ for children, young adults and adults. The Mental Capacity Act (MCA) 2005 has enshrined in statute the presumption that adults and young people aged 16 years and older (further to section 8 Family Law Reform Act 1969) will have decision-making capacity unless they have some permanent or temporary *impairment of, or a disturbance in the functioning of, the mind or brain* (MCA 2005, s2 (1)) which renders them unable to make a decision about a particular issue. The position for children aged under 16 is different. The case of *Gillick* v *West Norfolk and Wisbech AHA* [1986] established that children *may* have capacity to consent to treatment, providing that they fully understand the implications both of having and not having the treatment, and are able to demonstrate that they can both recall this information and make their decision known (GMC 2007).

If the patient lacks decision-making capacity (according to the provisions of the MCA 2005), treatment may still be given providing:

- it is in the patient's best interests (MCA 2005, s (5) (b) (ii), and
- the patient has not made a valid advance decision refusing that treatment (MCA 2005, s (24) (1)).

It may sometimes be necessary for the court to make an order that treatment would be in the patient's interests and may therefore go ahead lawfully:

> *The substantive law is that a proposed operation is lawful if it is in the best interests of the patient, and unlawful if it is not. What is required from the court, therefore, is not an order giving approval to the operation, so as to make lawful that which would otherwise be unlawful. What is required from the court is rather an order which establishes by judicial process … whether the proposed operation is in the best interests of the patient and therefore lawful, or not in the patient's best interests and therefore unlawful.* (Lord Oakbrook in *F* v *West Berkshire Health Authority (Mental Health Act Commission intervening)* [1989]: 557)

Nurses have the same duty of care when working with patients who lack decision-making capacity as they do when caring for those able to provide valid consent to treatment, and the standard set out in the 'Bolam test' will apply. Abhorrent as the necessity for such legislation might seem, the MCA 2005, section 44 recognises the vulnerability of people with impaired capacity to make decisions, and sets out the criminal offences of ill-treatment or neglect of a person without capacity.

Refusal of consent

If an adult (over 18 years in the UK) with decision-making capacity refuses consent, then treatment may not go ahead, even if those caring for that patient consider their decision to be foolish or irrational or the refusal results in the patient's death (e.g., *Re T (An Adult: Refusal of Medical Treatment)* [1992], *Kings College Hospital NHS Foundation Trust* v *C and V* [2015]). This may be very difficult for health care professionals to accept, but the right to self-determination is so important that sometimes this must supersede even *the principle of sanctity of human life* (Lord Goff in *Airedale NHS Trust* v *Bland* [1993]: 864) (to be referred to as: *Airedale* v *Bland* [1993]). In one well publicised case (Bowcott 2015; Clarke-Billings 2015; Coleman 2015) a woman exercised her right to refuse life-sustaining treatment on the grounds that she was no longer able to live a life that *sparkles* (*Kings College Hospital NHS Foundation Trust* v *C and V* [2015] para 8). MacDonald MJ: *A patient with capacity has the right to decide whether or not to accept treatment … based on the things that are important to her, in keeping with her own personality and system of values and without conforming to society's expectation of what constitutes the 'normal' decision in this situation (if such a thing exists). As a capacitous individual C is, in respect of her own body and mind, sovereign* (*Kings College Hospital NHS Foundation Trust* v *C and V* [2015] para 97).

For children and young adults (those aged between 16 and 18 years) the position is different. Providing they have decision-making capacity they may consent to treatment, even if their parents (or those with parental responsibility for them) do not consent to the treatment. However, if the child or young person refuses to consent, then the treatment may lawfully go ahead providing their parents, those with parental responsibility or the court do consent (*Re W (A Minor) (Medical Treatment: Court's Jurisdiction)* [1992]).

Activity 8.5   *Reflection*

Think about the previous paragraphs relating to refusal of consent, and the scenario describing Amy's refusal of treatment by intravenous infusion of antibiotics. Have you ever been in a situation where a patient has refused to consent to treatment?

- How did this make you feel at the time? Were you tempted/did you attempt to make the patient change his or her mind?
- How do you think the patient felt about his or her decision?
- What makes you think that? Why do you think the patient made that decision?
- How did the patient's family and friends respond?
- What impact did this refusal have on your care of the patient?
- How did the matter conclude?
- How would you manage a situation like this in the future?

As this activity is based on your own observations, there is no outline answer at the end of this chapter.

In reflecting on Activity 8.5, you may have considered how difficult it is for health care professionals to accept a patient's decision to refuse treatment, e.g., when they know that treatment will relieve a patient's pain. Therefore, it is possible that professionals may try to influence the patient to change their decision. Some family members may want treatment regardless, as they truly believe it will save the patient's life. There are many other ways of analysing this, but what is important in all this is to do what is best for the patient – to act in the best interest of the patient.

Legal consideration of the sanctity of life

When individuals approach the end of their life, they may not be able to fulfil their holistic care needs. Their illness may bring with it severe pain, cognitive decline or other symptoms that make it difficult for them either to engage with or enjoy their usual daily activities. Their family and friends may find it increasingly difficult to watch the person they love deteriorate and possibly suffer.

You may find that managing symptoms is difficult for some patients, and they find their condition intolerable. They may ask: 'Is a life like this worth living?' This is a difficult question and confronts one of the fundamental principles of our society – that human life is sacred, and should be protected at all costs.

Activity 8.6   *Critical thinking*

Now, return to the start of this chapter and re-read the scenario relating to Amy, imagining she is one of your patients. Consider the following questions:

- How do you feel about Amy's decision? How easy is it to accept?
- What might be the impact on Amy's family, and her relationship with them?
- What is the potential effect on Amy's relationship with members of care staff?
- What is your role in supporting Amy and her family?

As this activity is based on your own observations, there is no outline answer at the end of this chapter.

The taking, or otherwise prematurely ending, of a life is considered so abhorrent that our society reserves its most severe sanctions for those who breach it. A conviction for murder – where the accused intended to kill or very seriously injure – brings with it a mandatory sentence of life imprisonment. Even where someone caused death without intending to do so and is found guilty of manslaughter, the court may still impose a sentence of life imprisonment.

In your reflection in Activity 8.6 your patient was able to make an informed decision to refuse ongoing medical treatment. The case of *Airedale* v *Bland* [1993] required the House of Lords (at that time the highest Court of Appeal, a role subsequently assumed by the Supreme Court in 2009: Slapper and Kelly 2015) to consider some challenging questions relating to withdrawing treatment, the sanctity of life and the lawfulness of acting in any way other than to preserve life for a person who was not able to make an informed decision about ongoing medical treatment.

Case study

Anthony Bland was 17 years old when he was involved in what has come to be known as the 'Hillsborough disaster'. He was a Liverpool FC supporter and, on 15 April 1989, had travelled to the Hillsborough football ground for a semi-final of the FA Cup between Liverpool FC and Nottingham Forest FC. More than 90 supporters of both teams died after a catastrophic crush developed. Anthony received serious injuries to his chest, and as a result his brain was deprived of oxygen, resulting in severe injury.

By the autumn of 1992 Anthony had been in what was then known as a 'persistent vegetative state' (PVS) for more than three years, with no prospect of recovery (this is now more generally referred to as a vegetative state (VS): Airedale v Bland [1993]; W (by her litigation friend B) v M (by her litigation friend the Official Solicitor) and others [2011]). His condition meant that, although he could breathe without assistance, all higher-level brain functions had been permanently destroyed. Anthony had no sensory or cognitive awareness, and other than breathing, he required assistance with every bodily function. He was fed via a nasogastric tube.

Both the doctors treating Anthony and his family were of the opinion that it was inappropriate for his treatment to continue. The health authority made an application to the court for a declaration that withdrawal of all life-sustaining support (including artificial ventilation, hydration and nutrition) could be done lawfully so that Mr Bland could die as peacefully and with as much dignity as possible. At first instance the judge granted the declarations, but the Official Solicitor appealed, arguing that a withdrawal of treatment breached the doctors' duty of care to Mr Bland and would also incur criminal liability.

The final appeal by Airedale NHS Trust was heard at the House of Lords in December 1992, and a number of fundamental issues were considered, including:

- Must a patient's life be preserved by all medical means, regardless of the circumstances?
- What is the difference between an act that will hasten death and withdrawal of life-sustaining treatment?

This tragic case, and the deeply moving report, provide useful clarification in a number of key areas.

Activity 8.7   *Critical thinking*

Read this section of Lord Goff's judgement (*Airedale* v *Bland* [1993]: 873) and, before reading the next section of this chapter, summarise the points raised:

[A]rtificial feeding is, in a case such as the present, no different from life support by a ventilator, and as such can lawfully be discontinued when it no longer fulfils any therapeutic purpose. To me, the crucial point in which I found myself differing from Mr Munby [barrister acting for the Official Solicitor, and opposing the withdrawal of treatment] was that I was unable to accept his treating the discontinuance of artificial feeding in the present case as equivalent to cutting a mountaineer's rope, or severing the air pipe of a deep sea diver. Once it is recognised, as I believe it must be, that the true question is not whether the doctor should take a course in which he will actively kill his patient, but rather whether he should continue to provide his patient with medical treatment or care which, if continued, will prolong his life, then, as I see it, the essential basis of Mr Munby's submissions disappears.

continued ...

> Now read this earlier section (*Airedale* v *Bland* [1993]: 867) and, before reading the next section of this chapter, summarise the points raised here:
>
> *The doctor who is caring for such a patient cannot, in my opinion, be under an absolute obligation to prolong his life by any means available to him, regardless of the quality of the patient's life. Common humanity requires otherwise, as do medical ethics and good medical practice accepted in this country and overseas. As I see it, the doctor's decision whether or not to take any such step must (subject to his patient's ability to give or withhold his consent) be made in the best interests of the patient. It is this principle too which, in my opinion, underlies the established rule that a doctor may, when caring for a patient who is, for example, dying of cancer, lawfully administer painkilling drugs despite the fact that he knows that an incidental effect of that application will be to abbreviate the patient's life. Such a decision may properly be made as part of the care of the living patient, in his best interests; and, on this basis, the treatment will be lawful. Moreover, where the doctor's treatment of his patient is lawful, the patient's death will be regarded in law as exclusively caused by the injury or disease to which his condition is attributable.*
>
> *A summary of the points will be given in the next section of this chapter.*

In relation to the judgement in Activity 8.7, the House of Lords provided some important clarification. You may have identified some of these when completing the activity:

1. Artificially administered hydration and nutrition are treatments and may lawfully be withdrawn or withheld if:

   a. they are no longer serving a therapeutic purpose or
   b. would no longer serve a therapeutic purpose and
   c. this would be in the patient's best interests.

2. If withdrawing or withholding artificial hydration and nutrition results in the shortening of a patient's life, then it is not the withdrawal of treatment that will have caused the death, but the underlying condition – for example, cancer or severe brain injury.
3. Such a withdrawal of treatment is regarded very differently in law to any act such as an overdose of analgesia that is deliberately intended either to end life or hasten death. This would be an unlawful killing.
4. However, it may be lawful to administer analgesia that is intended to act as palliative symptom control, even if an associated effect of this is to shorten the patient's life.
5. There is no legal obligation to continue treatment where the quality of a patient's life is poor and there is no prospect of recovery.

Careful reading of these points should help you to understand the legal principles underpinning guidelines for end of life care. The law does not provide for indiscriminate withdrawal, but instead makes very clear that feeding or hydration by artificial means should end only when they are providing no therapeutic purpose and to do so would be in the patient's best interests. The General Medical Council (2010) has provided detailed guidelines for practice.

Each case should be considered on an individual basis, and the House of Lords ruled that consideration of best interests will usually require that treatment is given. However, respect must be given to the principle of self-determination. Where a patient has decision-making capacity the patient may refuse to consent to any treatment:

> *for any reason, rational or irrational, or for no reason at all, even where that decision may lead to his or her own death.*
> (*Re MB (Medical Treatment)*) [1997]: 432)

This means that, even where health care professionals consider a potentially life-saving treatment to be in a patient's best interests, providing the patient has capacity, the patient is under no obligation to accept that treatment. *Airedale* v *Bland* [1993] predated the MCA 2005, and the provisions of this Act now shape the decision-making process for patients who no longer have decision-making capacity. You will recall the test for determining decision-making capacity from earlier in this chapter, and that there will be a presumption of decision-making capacity unless there is proof to the contrary (MCA 2005). So, assuming that the necessary assessment of capacity has been performed, and it has been concluded that your patient does not have capacity, how are treatment decisions at the end of life made?

Decision-making in end of life care where patients lack capacity

Where the patient lacks decision-making capacity, there are a number of alternative ways in which decisions can be made on the patient's behalf. The patient may have made a valid advance decision to refuse a specified treatment (ADRT) should the need for it arise when the patient no longer has capacity to make decisions (MCA 2005, s24). If health care professionals reasonably believe that an applicable and valid ADRT exists, they will be protected from legal liability for withdrawing or withholding treatment (e.g., breach of duty in negligence). However, a number of conditions must be satisfied for a valid ADRT (Department for Constitutional Affairs 2007):

1. The person making the advance decision (you may also see this referred to as an 'advance directive') must have mental capacity and be aged 18 or over at the time the decision was made.
2. The decision must specify treatment that the individual would like to refuse at a point when he or she no longer has decision-making capacity.
3. The decision must specify details of the treatment and the circumstances in which the patient would like to refuse it.
4. Any decision to refuse life-sustaining treatment must be in writing (make clear that the decision must still stand even if that individual's life is at risk), be signed and witnessed.

It is important to note that, whilst there is legal provision for patients to refuse treatment in advance, other than an obligation for professionals to respect (where possible) the patient's previously stated preferences (*Aintree University Hospitals NHS Foundation Trust* v *James* [2013]) (to be referred to as: *Aintree* v *James* [2013]), there is generally no allied right to demand treatment in advance (*R (on the application of Burke)* v *General Medical Council* [2006]).

In addition to, or instead of, an ADRT, patients may have created a lasting power of attorney (LPA) (MCA 2005, s10) giving another person authority to make decisions on their behalf once they have lost the capacity to make decisions. Although there is no facility for patients to specify what treatment they would choose should they lose capacity, this is something that they would have discussed with their LPA(s). The LPA(s) should use that information to guide decision making on behalf of the patient who no longer has capacity. The Court of Protection also has authority under the MCA (2005, s16) to appoint a deputy to make decisions for a patient who does not have capacity.

In the absence of all of these, doctors may provide any treatment they consider to be in the patient's best interests (MCA 2005, s5). If there is any disagreement between medical opinion and the views of the patient's family and friends, the usual course of action is for the hospital to apply to the Court of Protection for a declaration that the proposed treatment can go ahead (MCA 2005, s15). Any decision will be made in the patient's interests, and should as far as possible take into account what is known of the patient's wishes whilst they had capacity.

Other issues deliberated by the House of Lords in the case of *Airedale* v *Bland* [1993] included the principle of the sanctity of human life. It was held that there is no obligation to preserve a patient's life by medical means, regardless of the individual circumstances. Indeed, in Lord Goff's opinion, the withdrawal of medical support, such as artificial nutrition, hydration and ventilation, should be considered in the same way as any other medical treatment. If continuing with the treatment is no longer in the patient's best interests, then it will not be a breach of duty to discontinue treatment (this summary refers to lines 1–4 of Lord Goff's judgement, as referred to in Activity 8.7).

Lord Goff went on to clarify the law in relation to discontinuing medical treatment that is no longer in the patient's best interests. He asserted that this is fundamentally different to committing an act with the intention of shortening a patient's life (this summary refers to lines 5–12 of Lord Goff's judgement, as referred to in Activity 8.7), which would be unlawful. Therefore administration of medication with the intention of relieving pain would be lawful, even if it does have the secondary effect of shortening the patient's life. However, administration of analgesia with the intention of hastening death would be unlawful. The key difference is the intention behind the act.

The House of Lords made it clear that a decision to discontinue treatment could only be made after very careful consideration, and that a declaration from the Court of Protection would be necessary before artificial hydration or nutrition could lawfully be withheld or withdrawn from a patient in a VS. Since then, more recent guidance on applications for discontinuing treatment was issued by the Court of Protection in the case of *W (by her litigation friend B)* v *M (by her litigation friend the Official Solicitor) and others* [2011] (to be referred to as: *W* v *M* 2011).

Case study: *W* v *M* [2011]

In February 2003 Mary was aged 43 and she became unwell at home the night before she was due to go on a skiing trip with her partner, Simon. She complained of a headache and went to bed early. Simon discovered her in a drowsy and confused state. Mary quickly deteriorated and was taken to hospital, where she was found to be suffering from viral encephalitis. She went into a coma, and when she eventually emerged, was diagnosed as being in a VS as the result of extensive and permanent brain damage caused by the virus. From that point she required 24-hour assistance with all her needs, was doubly incontinent, and since April 2003 had been fed via a gastrostomy tube. Mary was also immobile. By the end of 2006, clinicians treating her at a specialist rehabilitation unit were of the view that there was unlikely to be any further improvement in her condition. By the time the case was heard in 2011, Mary had flexion contractures in the ankles, knees, hips and elbows.

On 16 January 2007, Mary's family and Simon made an application to the High Court Family Division for a ruling that Mary lacked capacity to make decisions about her medical care, and that it would be lawful to withhold and discontinue all life-sustaining treatment, including artificial hydration and nutrition. Although Simon reported that Mary had discussed with him the issue of ongoing treatment in such a situation, she had not written an advance directive, and there was no other evidence to support this.

Over the next two or three years there were a number of assessments of Mary's level of consciousness. Although she was initially thought to be in a VS, subsequent review by another expert suggested that her level of consciousness was higher than originally thought. In fact, her condition better fitted the criteria for someone in a minimally conscious state (MCS) rather than VS, and with intensive rehabilitation it was thought that Mary might recover further. However, despite five months of intensive rehabilitation, she failed to make any further improvement and did not demonstrate any high-level functional responses to her environment.

She was admitted to a nursing home in February 2008. At this point, and as part of the ongoing legal process, Mary was assessed again by a different expert. This assessment found that, although her condition was variable, there was no evidence that any aspect of Mary's life gave her satisfaction, pleasure, discomfort or pain. This new assessment placed Mary at the lowest end of MCS. It was the expert's opinion that it would be appropriate to withdraw life-sustaining treatment in order that Mary might die with dignity. Mary's family therefore decided to continue with the application, which was transferred to the new Court of Protection in February 2010. The two experts assessing Mary agreed that she remained in an MCS, with her responses less consistent than they had been previously. However, they disagreed over the question of withdrawing artificial hydration and nutrition.

In order to protect confidentiality, only initials are given in the case report. 'Mary' and 'Simon' are pseudonyms.

It is clear from the case report that over the years Mary and Simon had shared conversations about their wishes should they find themselves in such a tragic situation. Unfortunately these were never formalised by making a valid ADRT (MCA 2005, ss24–26). So, although Simon could use these discussions to help guide Mary's day-to-day care, it was not sufficient to allow a withdrawal of artificial hydration and nutrition. Therefore, given Mary's lack of capacity, and the absence of a valid ADRT, the court was required to determine whether it was in Mary's best interests (as per MCA 2005, s4) to withdraw and withhold all life-sustaining treatment, including artificial nutrition and hydration (*W*v *M* [2011]).

In order to establish what was in Mary's best interests, the court adopted a balance sheet approach that had been advocated in an earlier case (*Re A (Medical Treatment: Male Sterilisation)* [2000]). This approach evaluated the advantages of withdrawing treatment as opposed to continuing with it, taking into consideration factors other than those that are purely medical, including *emotional and other welfare issues* (*Re A* [2000]: 2000). The court also addressed a historic debate about the issue of 'intolerability', and whether that benchmark must be met before considering withdrawal of artificial hydration and nutrition to be in the patient's best interests. However, the view was that, rather than being a prerequisite for withdrawal of artificial hydration and nutrition, this should instead be considered as part of the balance sheet approach (*W*v *M* [2011]). The court also took into account how Mary's experience of life would be affected by necessary treatment (*NHS Trust* v *S* [2003]: 47) and other requirements, as per MCA 2005, s4, and the MCA 2005 Code of Practice (Department for Constitutional Affairs 2007).

In *W*v *M* [2011] the Court of Protection concluded that, although each case must be considered individually, it is likely that for individuals in a VS the balance will probably fall towards withdrawing treatment. For clinically unstable individuals in an MCS (MCA 2005, s4), best interests will determine the lawfulness of withdrawing life-sustaining treatment in those particular circumstances. Historically, the position is clearer for people such as Mary: although they are in an MCS, they are otherwise in a clinically stable condition. For these people, withdrawal of treatment was never considered to be in their best interests and would therefore be unlawful, and, with the necessary intent to kill, would be murder (*W*v *M* [2011]: 1328). However, a Court of Protection judgement published in 2015 suggests a shift away from that position (*Re N* [2015]). Mrs N was an independent and private woman who, by the end of 2015, was experiencing advanced symptoms of multiple sclerosis. She was reliant on others for all her personal and care needs. Although there was some argument that she was in a VS, the court accepted the evidence that she was in fact in an MCS. Prior to this point, and given the stability of Mrs N's condition, the approach taken in *W*v *M* [2011] would have meant that withdrawal of CANH would not have been in her best interests. Hayden MJ drew on case law such as *Aintree* v *James* [2013], where the Supreme Court confirmed that, while it will generally be in patients' best interests to act to preserve their life, it will not be in their best interests (Department for Constitutional Affairs 2007) to receive futile treatment. (The Supreme Court disagreed that a proposed treatment should be regarded as futile if it offered no potential for cure or palliation, stating instead that a treatment will not be futile if it offers some benefit to the patient, even if it *has no effect upon the underlying disease or disability* (*Aintree* v *James* [2013] para 43).) Lady Hale re-framed the question of *whether it would be lawful to withhold any or all … treatments* to a consideration instead of whether it would be in the patient's best interests for him to receive them (*Aintree* v *James* [2013] para 41). It was on this basis that Hayden MJ ruled that it would not be in Mrs N's best interests to continue receiving CANH, and that subject to specified conditions, it would therefore be unlawful for this treatment to be administered. Although the lack of a recognised advance decision had played a large part in the outcome of the *W v M* [2011] case, after hearing a range of evidence from Mrs N's family and others who knew her and had responsibility for her care, Hayden MJ was satisfied that *to force nutrition and hydration upon her is to fail to respect the person she is and the code by which she has lived her life* (*Re N* [2015] para 61).

Suicide and euthanasia

Until 1961 it was unlawful for someone to commit or attempt suicide, and until the Suicide Act 1961 was passed, anyone failing in an attempt to take his or her own life would face legal action. However, while it is no longer a crime to commit this act, it is still unlawful to assist a person who wants to bring his or her life to an end, as section 2 (1) Suicide Act 1961 makes clear:

> *A person who aids, abets, counsels or procures the suicide of another, or an attempt by another to commit suicide, shall be liable on conviction on indictment to imprisonment for a term not exceeding fourteen years.*

Despite a number of recent cases (*Pretty v UK* [2002]; *Nicklinson, R. (on the application of) v Ministry of Justice* [2012]), there has been no shift in the legal position relating to assisted suicide, or euthanasia. Whereas some commentators would argue there is nothing ethically to distinguish between withdrawing or withholding treatments and acts deliberately intended to hasten someone's death, the law is very clear on the difference (*Airedale v Bland* [1993]). It remains unlawful to commit such an act, regardless of the motives behind it.

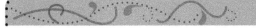

Chapter summary

This chapter has explored the law as it relates to some of the difficult decisions that are made at the end of life. As the focus of care shifts from recovery to palliation many people are uncomfortable with the idea of either withdrawing or withholding active treatment. We have explored the issue of consent and emphasised the importance of informed consent. Health care decisions at the end of life often involve a complex interplay of legal, ethical and professional issues that require careful consideration by the multidisciplinary team and may even require a court declaration before care can continue. As a student health care professional you will find it very useful to understand the basis of these decisions, even if you disagree with them, but you will not be expected to make them on your own. Here are some useful summary points for your guidance:

1. Health care professionals have a legal duty to provide care for their patients.
2. The standard of care will be judged against what is regarded (by other professionals) as acceptable at the time of treatment.

continued ...

3. Patients have a right to refuse treatment or other therapeutic interventions.
4. Treatment without a patient's consent will usually be unlawful.
5. When a patient does not have the capacity to make decisions, there are legal guidelines that health care professionals should follow.
6. It may be lawful either to withdraw or withhold life-sustaining treatment.
7. It will never be lawful to end another person's life deliberately, or assist that person to take his or her own life.

Activities: brief outline answers

Activity 8.2: Decision-making

Scenario 1

1. Does a duty of care exist? Yes, the neighbour principle in *Donoghue* v *Stevenson* [1932]. You could reasonably foresee that other people using the library could be affected by your acts or omissions. You therefore have a duty of care to them.
2. Has it been breached (either by doing something or failing to do something that a reasonable person would either have done or not done)? Would a 'reasonable person' (*Blyth* v *The Company of Proprietors of the Birmingham Waterworks* [1856]) throw a banana skin on to the floor? Probably not. A reasonable person would understand that there is a chance someone could slip on it and suffer injury.
3. Has harm been suffered? Yes – Hanna broke her wrist as a direct result of slipping on the banana skin.
4. Of a type that is reasonably foreseeable? Yes – this type of injury is reasonably foreseeable.

There is therefore likely to be liability in negligence in this scenario.

Scenario 2

1. Does a duty of care exist? Yes, the neighbour principle in *Donoghue* v *Stevenson* [1932]. You should reasonably foresee that by leaving the gate open the sheep might escape into the lane and therefore people using the lane, e.g., walkers, cyclists, motorists, could be affected by your omission. You therefore have a duty of care to them. You would also have a duty of care to the farmers as your failure to act is likely to affect them.
2. Has it been breached (either by doing something or failing to do something that a reasonable person would either have done or not done)? Would a 'reasonable person' (*Blyth* v *The Company of Proprietors of the Birmingham Waterworks* [1856]) leave a gate in the countryside open? No – and it is also a breach of the countryside code.
3. Has harm been suffered? Yes – the cyclists have suffered injuries, and their bikes have been damaged. The on-coming driver has incurred damage to their car, and may suffer subsequent psychological distress. The farmer has suffered damage to livestock.
4. Of a type that is reasonably foreseeable? Yes – this type of injury/harm is reasonably foreseeable.

There is therefore likely to be liability in negligence in this scenario.

Further reading

Cooke, J. (2011) *Law of Tort*, 10th edn. Harlow: Pearson Education.

This text is written specifically for the student. It provides a clear explanation of the main principles of tort law.

Herring, J. (2016) *Medical Law and Ethics*, 6th edn. Oxford: Oxford University Press.

An overview of medical law as it relates to ethical theory and the current social and health care context.

Mason, J.K. and Laurie, G.T. (2016) *Law and Medical Ethics*, 10th edn. Oxford: Oxford University Press.

An overview of medical law and ethical theory within the context of contemporary health care. Recent developments in the law are also explored.

Slapper, G. and Kelly, D. (2015) *The English Legal System 2015–2016*, 16th edn. London: Routledge.

A critical exploration of the origins and development of English law, and how it is applied in practice.

Taylor, H. (2013) Determining capacity to consent to treatment. *Nursing Times*, 109 (43): 12–14.

This article provides further information about an individual's right to choose, the legal meaning of the word 'consent' and the importance of gaining consent before treating a patient.

Taylor, H. (2013) What does consent mean in clinical practice? *Nursing Times*, 109 (44): 30–32.

This article considers the meaning of consent in practice and explores the conditions that must be satisfied for consent to be valid.

Taylor, H. (2015) Legal and ethical issues in end of life care: implications for primary health care. *Primary Healthcare*, 25 (4): 32–40.

This article provides further consideration of legal issues at the end of life, including the issue of administering treatment (such as analgesia and sedation) which may hasten a patient's death.

Wheeler, H. (2012) *Law, Ethics and Professional Issues for Nursing*. London: Routledge.

Useful websites

www.nhsiq.nhs.uk/improvement-programmes/long-term-conditions-and-integrated-care/end-of-life-care.aspx

A link to a range of resources published by NHS Improving Quality to support and inform end of life care.

www.gmc-uk.org/guidance/ethical_guidance/end_of_life_care.asp

General Medical Council guidance on end of life care.

www.nmc.org.uk/globalassets/sitedocuments/nmc-publications/nmc-code.pdf

Nursing and Midwifery Council Code: professional standards of practice and behaviour for nurses and midwives.

References

Adam, S.K. and Osborne, S. (2005) *Critical Care Nursing: Science and Practice*. Oxford: Oxford University Press.

Addington-Hall, J.M.(2007) *Research Methods in Palliative Care*. Oxford: Oxford University Press.

Aintree University Hospitals NHS Foundation Trust v James [2013] UKSC 67 (online). Available from: www.bailii.org.uk/cases/UKSC/2013/67.html (accessed 19 August 2016).

Airedale Hospital Trustees v *Bland* [1993] AC 789 (online). Available from: www.bailii.org/uk/cases/UKHL/17.pdf (accessed 1 September 2016).

Alzheimer's Disease International (2015) *The Global Impact of Dementia: An Analysis of Prevalence, Incidence, Costs and Trends*. London: Alzheimer's Disease International.

Andershed, B. (2006) Relatives in end-of-life care – part 1: a systematic review of the literature the five last years, January 1999–February 2004. *Journal of Clinical Nursing*, 15: 1158–1169.

Arbour, R. and Wiegland, D. (2014) Self-described nursing roles experienced during care of dying patients and their families: a phenomenological study. *Intensive and Critical Care Nursing*, 30: 211–218.

Aries, P. (1974) *Western Attitudes Towards Death: From the Middle Ages to the Present*. New York: Marion Boyars.

Astley-Pepper, M. (2005) Social erosion or isolation in palliative care. In: Nyatanga, B. and Astley-Pepper, M. (eds) *Hidden Aspects of Palliative Care*. London: Quay Books.

Beauchamp, T. and Childress, J. (2009) *Principles of Biomedical Ethics*, 6th edn. Oxford: Oxford University Press.

Bendorf, A., Kelly, P., Kerridge, I., McCaughan, G., Myerson, B., Stewart, C. and Pussell, B. (2013) An international comparison of the effect of policy shifts to organ donation following cardiocirculatory death (DCD) on donation rates after brain death (DBD) and transplantation rates. *PLOS One*, 8 (5): e62010.

Benjamin, M. and Curtis, J. (2010) *Ethics in Nursing: Cases, Principles and Reasoning*, 4th edn. Oxford: Oxford University Press.

Berry, J.W., Poortinga, Y.H., Segall, M.H. and Dasen, P.R. (1992) *Cross-cultural Psychology: Research and Applications*. Cambridge, MA: Cambridge University Press.

Berry, P. and Griffe, J. (2015) Planning for the actual death. In: Ferrell, B.R. and Coyle, N. (eds) *Oxford Textbook of Palliative Nursing*, 4th edn. Oxford: Oxford University Press, 515–531.

Bishop, A. and Scudder, J. (2001) *Nursing Ethics: Holistic Caring Practice.* Burlington, MA: Jones and Bartlett.

Blackhall, A., Hawkes, D., Hingley, A. and Wood, S. (2011) VERA framework: communicating with people who have dementia. *Nursing Standard,* 26 (10): 35–39.

Blyth v *The Company of Proprietors of the Birmingham Waterworks* [1856] 156 ER 1047 (online). Available from: Lexis®Library (accessed 1 September 2016).

Boa, S., Duncan, E.A.S., Haraldsdottir, E. and Wyke, S. (2014) Goal setting in palliative care: a structured review. *Progress in Palliative Care,* 22 (6): 326–333.

Bolam v *Friern Management Committee* [1957] 2 All ER 118 (online). Available from: Lexis®Library (accessed 19 August 2016).

Bolitho v *City and Hackney H.A.* [1997] 4 All ER 771 HL (online). Available from: www. bailii.org/ cgi-bin/markup.cgi?doc=/uk/cases/UKHL/ 1997/46.html&query=title+ (+Bolitho+ &method= boolean (accessed 19 August 2016).

Bowcott, O. (2015) Court grants woman right to die after 'losing her sparkle'. *The Guardian,* 2 December (online). Available from: www.theguardian.com/uk-news/2015/dec/02/court-grants-impulsive-self-centred-mother-permission-to-die (accessed 24 September 2016).

Brown, G. (2008) *The Living End: The Future of Death, Ageing and Immortality.* London: Macmillan.

Buglass, E. (2010) Grief and bereavement theories. *Nursing Standard,* 24 (41): 44–47.

Calanzani, N., Gomes, B. and Higginson, I.J. (2013) *Current and Future Needs for Hospice Care: An Evidence-Based Report.* London: Help the Hospices.

Carter, H., MacLeod, R., Brander, P. and McPherson, K. (2003) Living with a terminal illness: patients' priorities. *Journal of Advanced Nursing,* 45 (6): 611–620.

Cassidy v *Ministry of Health* [1951] 1 All ER 574 (online). Available from: Lexis®Library (accessed 1 September 2016).

Chan, D., Livingston, G., Jones, L. and Sampson, E.L. (2012) Grief reactions in dementia carers: a systematic review. *Geriatric Psychiatry,* 28: 1–17.

Chapman, L. (2009) Adapting the Liverpool Care Pathway for intensive care units. *European Journal of Palliative Care,* 16 (3): 116–118.

Chester v *Afshar* [2004] UKHL 41 (online). Available from: www.bailii.org/cgi-bin/markup. cgi?doc=/uk/cases/UKHL/2004/41.html&query=title+(+chester+)+and+title+(+v+)+and+title+(+afshar+)&method=boolean (accessed 1 September 2016).

Clark, J. (2003) Patient centered death: we need better, more innovative research on patients' views on dying. *British Medical Journal,* 327 (7408): 174–175.

Clarke, J. (2013) *Spiritual Care in Everyday Nursing Practice.* Basingstoke: Palgrave Macmillan.

Clarke-Billings, L. (2015) Woman, 50, wins right to refuse life-saving treatment because her 'sparkle' has gone. *The Telegraph,* 1 December (online). Available from: www.telegraph.co.uk/news/health/news/12027751/Woman-50-wins-right-to-refuse-life-saving-treatment-because-her-sparkle-has-gone.html (accessed 24 September 2016).

Cohen, S.L., Bewley, J.S., Ridley, S., Goldhill, D. and Members of The ICS Standards Committee (2003) *Guidelines for the Limitation of Treatment for Adults Requiring Intensive Care*. Intensive Care Society (online). Available from: www.ics.ac.uk/intensive_care_professional/standards_and_guidelines/limitation_of_treatment_2003 (accessed March 2011).

Coleman, C. (2015) Why a woman who lost her 'sparkle' was allowed to die. *BBC News*, 2 December (online). Available from: www.bbc.co.uk/news/uk-34985442 (accessed 24 September 2016).

Collins v *Wilcock* [1984] 3 All ER 374 (online). Available from: Lexis®Library (accessed 1 September 2016).

Commissioning Board Chief Nursing Officer and DH Chief Nursing Adviser (2012) *Compassion in Practice: Nursing, Midwifery and Care Staff: Our Vision and Strategy*. NHS Commissioning Board (online). Available from: www.england.nhs.uk/wp-content/uploads/2012/12/compassion-in-practice.pdf (accessed 10 March 2014).

Consumer Rights Act 2015 (c.15) (online). Available from: www.legislation.gov.uk/ukpga/2015/15/data.pdf (accessed 19 August 2016).

Coombs, M. and Long, T. (2008) Managing a good death in critical care: can health policy help? *Nursing in Critical Care*, 13 (4): 208–213.

Coombs, M.A., Addington-Hall, J. and Long-Sutehall, T. (2012) Challenges in transition from intervention to end of life care in intensive care: a qualitative study. *International Journal of Nursing Studies*, 49: 519–527.

Coombs, M., Darlington, A., Long-Sutehall, T. and Richardson, A. (2015) Transferring critically ill patients home to die: developing a clinical guidance document. *Nursing in Critical Care*, 20 (5): 264–270.

Covington, H. (2003) Caring presence: delineation of a concept for holistic nursing. *Journal of Holistic Nursing*, 21 (3): 301–317.

Criminal Justice Act 1988 (c.33) (online). Available from: www.legislation.gov.uk/ukpga/1988/33/data.pdf (accessed 1 September 2016).

Curtis, J.R. and Vincent, J. (2010) Ethics and end-of-life care for adults in the intensive care unit. *Lancet*, 376 (9749): 1347–1353.

Day, A., Haj-Bakri, S., Lubchansky, S. and Mehta, S. (2013) Sleep, anxiety and fatigue in family members of patients admitted to the intensive care unit: a questionnaire study. *Critical Care*, 17: R91.

De Souza, J. (2012) Calling in the palliative care team. In: Pettifer, A. and De Souza, J. (eds) *End-of-Life Nursing Care: A Guide for Best Practice*. London: Sage.

Deitz, J.H. (1981) *Rehabilitation Oncology*. Chichester: John Wiley and Sons.

Del Piccolo, L., Goss, C. and Zimmermann, C. (2006) Consensus finding on the appropriateness of provider responses to patient cues and concerns. *Journal of Patient Education and Counselling*, 61: 473–475.

Department for Constitutional Affairs (2007) *Mental Capacity Act 2005: Code of Practice*. London: The Stationery Office.

Department of Health (2000) *Comprehensive Critical Care: A Review of Adult Critical Care Services*. London: Department of Health.

Department of Health (2008) *End of Life Care Strategy: Promoting High Quality Care for All Adults at the End of Life*. London: Department of Health (online). Available from: www.gov.uk/government/uploads/system/uploads/attachment_data/file/497253/Mental-capacity-act-code-of-practice.pdf (accessed 1 September 2016).

Department of Health (2012) *Long Term Conditions Compendium of Information*, 3rd edn (online). Available from: www.gov.uk/government/uploads/system/uploads/attachment_data/file/216528/dh_134486.pdf (accessed 29 March 2017).

Department of Health (2016) *Our Commitment to You for End of Life Care*. Available from: www.gov.uk/government/uploads/system/uploads/attachment_data/file/536326/choice-response.pdf (accessed 31 August 2016).

Dixon, J., King, D. and Knapp, M. (2016) Advance care planning in England: is there an association with place of death? Secondary analysis of data from the National Survey of Bereaved People. *BMJ Supportive Palliative Care* (online). Available from: www.ncbi.nlm.nih.gov/pubmed/27312056 (accessed 21 January 2017).

Donoghue v *Stevenson* [1932] AC 562 (online). Available from: Lexis®Library (accessed 1 September 2016).

Duke, S. and Bennett, H. (2010) A narrative review of the published ethical debates in palliative care research and an assessment of their adequacy to inform research governance. *Palliative Medicine*, 24: 111–126.

Eide, H., Quera, V., Graugaard, P. and Finset, A. (2004) Physician–patient dialogue surrounding patients' expression of concern: applying sequence analysis to RIAS. *Social Science and Medicine*, 59 (1): 145–155.

F v *West Berkshire Health Authority (Mental Health Act Commission intervening)* [1989] 2 All ER 545 (online). Available from: Lexis®Library (accessed 21 July 2013).

Fagan v *Metropolitan Police Commissioner* [1968] 3 All ER 442 (online). Available from: Lexis®Library (accessed 1 September 2016).

Family Law Reform Act 1969 (c.46) (online). Available from: www.legislation.gov.uk/ukpga/1969/46/data.pdf (accessed 1 September 2016).

Field, N.P. and Filanosky, C. (2009) Continuing bonds: risk factors to complicated grief and adjustment to bereavement. *Death Studies*, 34 (1): 1–29.

Francis, R. (2013) *Report of the Mid Staffordshire NHS Foundation Trust Public Inquiry*. London: The Stationery Office.

Freud, S. (1917) *Mourning and Melancholia. The Standard Edition of the Complete Psychological Works of Sigmund Freud, Volume XIV (1914–1916): On the History of the Psycho-Analytical Movement, Papers on Metapsychology and Other Works*. London: Hogarth Press and Institute of Psycho-Analysis, 237–258.

Furze, G. (2015) Goal setting: a key skill for person-centred care. *Practice Nursing*, 26 (5): 241–244.

Gallagher, A. and Hodge, S. (2012) *Ethics, Law and Professional Issues: A Practice-Based Approach for Health Care Professionals*, 2nd edn. Basingstoke: Palgrave Macmillan.

Gallagher, A., Bousso, R., McCarthy, J., Kohlen, H., Andrews, T., Paganini, M., Abu-El-Noor, N., Cox, A., Haas, M., Arber, Abu-El-Noor, M., Baliza, M. and Padilha, G. (2015) Negotiated reorientating: a grounded theory of nurses' end-of-life decision-making in the intensive care unit. *International Journal of Nursing Studies*, 52: 794–803.

General Medical Council (2007) *0–18 Years: Guidance for All Doctors* (online). Available from: www.gmc-uk.org/static/documents/content/0_18_years.pdf (accessed 19 August 2016).

General Medical Council (2010) *Treatment and Care Towards The End of Life: Good Practice in Decision Making* (online). Available from: www.gmc-uk.org/static/documents/ content/Treatment_and_care_towards_the_end_of_life_-_English_1015.pdf (accessed 1 September 2016).

Gibbs, G. (1988) *Learning by Doing: A Guide to Teaching and Learning Methods*. Further Education Unit. Oxford: Oxford Polytechnic.

Gilbert, P. (ed.) (2013) *Spirituality and End of Life Care*. Hove: Pavillion Publishing.

Gillick v *West Norfolk and Wisbech AHA* [1986] AC 112 (online). Available from: www.bailii.org/uk/cases/UKHL/1985/7.pdf (accessed 1 September 2016).

Goldberg, D.P., Jenkins, L., Millar, T. and Faragher, E.B. (1993) The ability of trainee general practitioners to identify psychosocial distress among their patients. *Psychological Medicine*, 23: 185–193.

Goldberg, D.S., French, B., Abt, P.L., Olthoff, K. and Shaked, A. (2014) Superior survival using living donors and donor-recipient matching using a novel living donor risk index. *Hepatology* 60.5: 1717–1726.

Goodhead, A. (2010) A textual analysis of memorials written by bereaved individuals and families in a hospice context. *Mortality*, 15 (14): 323–339.

Gott, M., Seymour, J., Bellamy, G. and Ahmedzai, S. (2004) Older people's views about home as a place of care at the end of life. *Palliative Medicine*, 18: 460–467.

(The) Guardian (2016). Available from: www.theguardian.com/world/2016/jul/14/several-killed-after-lorry-drives-into-crowd-in-nice-reports (accessed 3 April 2017).

Gysels, S.M., Evans, C. and Higginson, J. (2012) Patient, caregiver, health professional and researcher views and experiences of participating in research at end of life: a critical interpretive synthesis of the literature. *Journal of Palliative Medicine*, (12): 123.

Gysels, M., Evans, C.J., Lewis, P., Spech, P., Hamia, B., Preston, N.J., Grande, G.E., Short, V., Todd, C.J. and Higginson, I.J. (2013) MORECare research methods guidance development: recommendations for ethical issues in palliative and end of life care research. *Palliative Medicine*, 27 (10): 908–917.

Halsbury's Laws of England (2010) *Negligence,* vol. 78, 5th edn (online). Available from: Lexis®Library (accessed 19 August 2016).

Halsbury's Laws of England (2011) *Negligence and Duties Owed to Patients,* vol. 74, 5th edn (online). Available from: Lexis®Library (accessed 19 August 2016).

Halsbury's Laws of England (2015) *Tort,* vol. 97, 5th edn (online). Available from: Lexis®Library (accessed 19 August 2016).

Hawker, S., Payne, S., Kerr, C., Hardey, M. and Powell, J. (2002) Appraising the evidence: reviewing disparate data systematically. *Qualitative Health Research,* 12 (9): 1284–1299.

Hawley, G. (2007) *Ethics in Clinical Practice.* Edinburgh: Pearson.

Health and Social Care Information Centre (2016) *Hospital Episode Statistics Adult Critical Care in England: April 2014 to March 2015.* Available from: http://content.digital.nhs.uk/catalogue/PUB19938/adul-crit-care-data-eng-apr-14-mar-15-rep.pdf (accessed 3 April 2017).

Humphrey, G.M. and Zimpfer, D.G. (2008) *Counselling for Grief and Bereavement,* 2nd edn. London: Sage.

Hunt, K.J., Shlomo, N. and Addington-Hall, J. (2014) End-of-life care and achieving preferences for place of death in England: results of a population-based survey using the VOICES-SF questionnaire. *Palliative Medicine* (online). Available from: www.ncbi.nlm.nih.gov/pubmed/24292157 (accessed 21 January 2017).

Independent Review of the Liverpool Care Pathway (2013) *More Care, Less Pathway: A Review of the Liverpool Care Pathway* (online). Available from: www.gov.uk/ government/uploads/system/uploads/attachment_data/file/212450/Liverpool_Care_Pathway.pdf (accessed 19 August 2016).

Intensive Care National Audit and Research Centre (2010) *CMP Case Mix and Outcome Summary Statistics* (online). Available from: www.icnarc.org/documents/summary%20statistics%20 2008–9.pdf (accessed 7 February 2014).

Intensive Care Society (2003) *Guidelines for Limitations of Treatment for Adults Requiring Intensive Care.* London: Intensive Care Society.

Intensive Care Society (2011) *End of Life Care for Adults* (online). Available from: www.nice.org.uk/guidance/qualitystandards/endoflifecare/home.jsp (accessed 26 January 2012).

Kastenbaum, R.J. (2011) *Death, Society and Human Experience.* Abingdon: Routledge.

Kings College Hospital NHS Foundation Trust v *C and V* [2015] EWCOP 59 (online). Available from: www.bailii.org/ew/cases/EWCOP/2015/80.html (accessed 19 August 2016).

Kisvetrová, H., Klugar, M. and Kabelka, L. (2013) Spiritual support interventions in nursing care for patients suffering death anxiety in the final phase of life. *International Journal of Palliative Nursing,* 19 (12): 599–605.

Khan, N.F., Harrison, S., Rose, P.W., Ward, A. and Evans, J. (2012) Interpretation and acceptance of the term 'cancer survivor': a United Kingdom based qualitative study. *European Journal of Cancer Care,* 21: 177–186.

Klass, D., Silverman, P.R. and Nickman, S.L. (1996) *Continuing Bonds: A New Understanding of Grief.* Philadelphia, PA: Taylor and Francis.

Koffman, J. and Richardson, H. (2011) Embracing diversity at the end of life. In: Oliviere, D., Monroe, B. and Payne, S. (eds) *Death, Dying and Social Difference.* Oxford: Oxford University Press.

Kroeber, A.L. and Kluckholn, C. (1952) *A Critical Review of Concepts and Definitions.* Vol. 47. Cambridge, MA: Peabody Museum of Archeology and Ethnology.

Kübler-Ross, E. (1973) *On Death and Dying.* London: Routledge.

Lawson, J. (2001) Gaining and maintaining consent: ethical concerns raised in a study of dying patients. *Qualitative Health Research*, 11 (5): 693–705.

Leadership Alliance for the Care of Dying People (2014) *One Chance to Get It Right* (online). Available from: www.gov.uk/government/uploads/system/uploads/attachment_data/file/323188/One_chance_to_get_it_right.pdf (accessed 31 August 2016).

Lee, S. and Kristjanson, L. (2003) Human research ethics committees in palliative care research. *International Journal on Palliative Nursing*, 9 (1): 13–18.

Levine, M.E. (1971) Holistic nursing. *Nursing Clinics of North America*, 6 (2): 253–264.

Locke, E.A. and Latham, G.P. (2002) Building a practically useful theory of goal setting and task motivation. *American Psychologist*, 57 (9): 705–717.

Long-Sutehall, T., Willis, H., Palmer, R., Ugboma, D., Addington-Hall, J. and Coombs, M. (2011) Negotiated dying: a grounded theory of how nurses shape withdrawal of treatment in hospital critical care units. *International Journal of Nursing Studies*, 48: 1466–1474.

Lunney, J.R., Lynn, J. and Hogan, C. (2002) Profiles of older Medicare decedents. *Journal of the American Geriatric Society*, 50 (6): 1108–1112.

Lusardi, P., Jodka, P., Stambovsky, M., Stadnicki, B., Babb, B., Plouffe, D., Doubleday, N., Pizlak, Z., Walles, K. and Montonye, M. (2011) The going home initiative: getting critical care patients home with hospice. *Critical Care Nurse*, 31 (5): 46–57.

McAree, S.J. and Doherty, P.A. (2010) A survey regarding physician preferences in end-of-life practices in intensive care across Scotland. *Journal of the Intensive Care Society*, 11 (3): 182–185.

McCallum, A. and McConigley, R. (2013) Nurses' perceptions of caring for dying patients in an open critical care unit: a descriptive exploratory study. *International Journal of Palliative Nursing*, 19 (1): 25–30.

McEvoy, L. and Duffy, A. (2008) Holistic practice: a concept analysis. *Nurse Education in Practice*, 8 (16): 412–419.

McGlade, D., McClenahan, C. and Pierscionek, B. (2014). Pro-donation behaviours of nursing students from the four countries of the UK. *PLOS One* 9.3: e91405.

McLeod, A. (2014) Nurses' views of the causes of ethical dilemmas during treatment cessation in the ICU: a qualitative study. *British Journal of Neuroscience Nursing*, 10 (3): 131–137.

Macmillan Cancer Support (2013) *Throwing Light on the Consequences of Cancer and Its Treatment* (online). Available from: www.macmillan.org.uk/documents/aboutus/research/researchand evaluationreports/throwinglightontheconsequencesofcanceranditstreatment.pdf (accessed 24 November 2016).

Macmillan Cancer Support (2014) *A Competency Framework for Nurses, Caring for Patients Living with and Beyond Cancer* (online). Available from: www.macmillan.org.uk/_images/competence-framework-for-nurses_tcm9-297835.pdf (accessed 24 November 2016).

Maddams, J., Utley, M. and Møller, H. (2012) Projections of cancer prevalence in the United Kingdom 2010–2040. *British Journal of Cancer*, 107 (7): 1195–1202.

Maguire, P., Faulkner, A., Booth, K., Elliot, C. and Hillier, V.F. (1996) Helping cancer patients disclose their concerns. *European Journal of Cancer*, 32: 78–81.

Martin, S. and Bristowe, K. (2015) Last offices: nurses' experiences of the process and their views about involving significant others. *International Journal of Palliative Nursing*, 21 (4): 173–178.

Matsumoto, D. and Juang, L. (2012) *Culture and Psychology*, 5th edn. New York: Cengage Learning.

Matzo, M., Sherman, D., Lo, K., Egan, K., Grant, M. and Rhome, A. (2003) Strategies for teaching loss, grief and bereavement. *Nurse Educator*, 28 (2): 71–76.

Mehrabian, A. (1967) Significance of posture and position in the communication of attitude and status relationships. *Psychological Bulletin*, 71 (5): 359–372.

Mental Capacity Act 2005 (c.9) (online). Available from: www.legislation.gov.uk/ ukpga/2005/9/ data.pdfs/ukpga_20050009_en.pdf (accessed 19 August 2019).

Molter, N.C. (1979) Needs of relatives of critically ill patients: a descriptive study. *Heart and Lung*, 8 (2): 332–339.

Montgomery v *Lanarkshire Health Board* [2015] (online). Available from: www.bailii.org/uk/cases/ UKSC/2015/11.pdf (accessed 1 September 2016).

Mosby's Medical Dictionary (2009), 8th edn. St Louis, MO: Elsevier.

National Council for Palliative Care (NCPC) (2015) *Care after Death Guidance*, 2nd edn. London: Hospice UK.

National End of Life Care Intelligence Network (2012) (online). Available from: www. endoflifecare-intelligence.org.uk/resources/publications/ (accessed 3 April 2017).

National Institute for Health and Care Excellence (2013) *End of Life Care for Adults Quality Standard* (online). Available from: www.nice.org.uk/guidance/qs13 (accessed 15 November 2016).

National Institute for Health and Care Excellence (2015) *Care of Dying Adults in the Last Days of Life* (online). Available from: www.nice.org.uk/guidance/ng31 (accessed 20 August 2016).

National Institute for Health and Care Excellence (2016) *Organ Donation for Transplantation: Improving Donor Identification and Consent Rates for Deceased Organ Donation*. Available from: www.nice.org.uk/guidance/cg135/chapter/1-recommendations#seeking-consent-to-organ-donation (accessed 3 April 2017).

Nazarko, L. (2016) Organ donation: the gift of life at the point of death. *British Journal of Nursing*, 25 (6): 290.

NHS Blood and Transplant (2016) (online). Available from: www.nhsbt.nhs.uk/ (accessed 3 April 2017).

NHS Improving Quality (2015) *The Route to Success in End of Life Care: Achieving Quality for People with Learning Disabilities* (online). Available from: www.nhsiq.nhs.uk/resource-search/ publications/eolc-rts-learning-disabilities.aspx (accessed 21 August 2016).

NHS Trust v *S* [2003] EWHC 365 (Fam) (online). Available from: www.bailii.org/cgi-bin/ format.cgi?doc=/ew/cases/EWHC/Fam/2003/365.html&query=(title:(+NHS+))+AND+(title: (+Trust+))+AND+(title:(+v+))+AND+(title:(+S+)) (accessed 1 September 2016).

Nicklinson, R. (on the application of) v *Ministry of Justice* [2012] EWHC 2381 (Admin) (online). Available from: www.bailii.org/cgi-bin/markup.cgi?doc=/ew/cases/EWHC/Admin/2012/2381. html&query=Nicklinson&method=boolean (accessed 1 September 2016).

Nicol, J. (2015) *Nursing Adults with Long Term Conditions.* London: Sage.

Nouwen, H.J. (1982) *In Memoriam.* Notre Dame, IN: Ave Maria Press.

Nursing and Midwifery Council (2010) *Standards for Pre-registration Nursing Education.* London: Nursing and Midwifery Council.

Nursing and Midwifery Council (2015) *The Code: Standards of Conduct, Performance and Ethics for Nurses and Midwives* (online). Available from: www.nmc.org.uk/globalassets/sitedocuments/nmc-publications/nmc-code.pdf (accessed 1 September 2016).

Nyatanga, B. (2008a) *Why Is It So Difficult to Die?* London: Quay Books.

Nyatanga, B. (2008b) Cultural competence: a noble idea in a changing world. *International Journal of Palliative Nursing,* 14 (7): 315.

Nyatanga, B. (2011) The pursuit of cultural competence: service accessibility and acceptability. *International Journal of Palliative Nursing,* 17 (5): 212–215.

Nyatanga, B. (2013) Attitudes to death: a time to pose difficult questions. *British Journal of Community Nursing,* 18 (10): 512.

Nyatanga, B. (2016) The essential pillars of palliative care. *British Journal of Community Nursing,* 21 (8): 418.

Nyatanga, B. and de Vocht, H. (2009) When last offices are more than just a white sheet. *British Journal of Nursing,* 18 (17): 1028.

Nyatanga, L. and Nyatanga, B. (2011) Death and dying. In: Birchenall, P. and Adam, N. (eds) *The Nursing Companion.* Basingstoke, Hampshire: Palgrave Macmillan.

Oberle, K. and Hughes, D. (2001) Doctors' and nurses' perceptions of ethical problems in end-of-life decisions. *Journal of Advanced Nursing,* 33 (6): 707–715.

Office for National Statistics (2011) *UK Census 2011* (online). Available from: www.ons.gov.uk/ons/guide-method/census/2011/census-data/index.html (accessed 6 February 2014).

Office for National Statistics (2012) *Religion in England and Wales* (online). Available from: www.ons.gov.uk/peoplepopulationandcommunity/culturalidentity/religion/articles/religionin englandandwales2011/2012-12-11 (accessed 15 November 2016).

Oliviere, D., Munroe, B. and Payne, S. (2011) *Death, Dying, and Social Differences,* 2nd edn. Oxford: Oxford University Press.

Pattison, N. (2008) Caring for patients after death. *Nursing Standard,* 22 (51): 48–56.

Pattison, N. (2011) End of life in critical care: an emphasis on care. *Nursing in Critical Care,* 16 (3): 113–115.

Pattison, N., Carr, S.M., Turnock, C. and Dolan, S. (2013) 'Viewing in slow motion': patients', families', nurses' and doctors' perspectives on end-of-life care in critical care. *Journal of Clinical Nursing,* 22: 1442–1454.

Pretty v *UK* [2002] 35 EHRR 1 (online). Available from: www.bailii.org/cgi-bin/markup. cgi?doc=/eu/cases/ECHR/2002/427.html&query=pretty&method=boolean (accessed 1 September 2016).

Prichep, D. (2013) *Death Cafes Breathe Life into Conversations About Death* (online). Available from: www.npr.org/2013/03/08/173808940/death-cafes-breathe-life-into-conversations-about-dying (accessed 10 January 2017).

Quested, B. and Rudge, T. (2003) Nursing care of dead bodies: a discursive analysis of last offices. *Journal of Advanced Nursing*, 41 (5): 553–560.

R (on the application of Burke) v *General Medical Council* [2006] 1 WLR 327 (online). Available from: Lexis®Library (accessed 1 September 2016).

Radbruch, L. (2011) Foreword. In: Oliviere, D., Monroe, B. and Payne, S. (eds) *Death, Dying and Social Difference*. Oxford: Oxford University Press.

Re A (Medical Treatment: Male Sterilisation) [2000] 1 FCR 193 (online). Available from: Lexis®Library (accessed 1 September 2016).

Re MB (Medical Treatment) [1997] EWCA Civ 3093 (online). Available from: www.bailii.org/cgi-bin/format.cgi?doc=/ew/cases/EWCA/Civ/1997/3093.html&query=(title:(+Re+))+AND+(title:(+MB+)) (accessed 1 September 2016).

Re N [2015] EWCOP 76 (online). Available from: www.bailii.org/ew/cases/EWCOP/2015/76.html (accessed 19 August 2016).

Re T (An Adult: Refusal of Medical Treatment) [1992] 4 All ER 649 (online). Available from: Lexis®Library (accessed 1 September 2016).

Re W (A Minor) (Medical Treatment: Court's Jurisdiction) [1992] 4 All ER 627 (online). Available from: Lexis®Library (accessed 1 September 2016).

Read, S. (2006) *Palliative Care for People with Learning Disabilities*. London: Quay Books.

Rogers, M.E. (1970) *An Introduction to the Theoretical Base of Nursing*. Philadelphia, PA: FA Davis.

Rosenblatt, P.C. (2015) Grief in small scale societies. In Murray Parkes, C., Laungani, P. and Young, B. (eds) *Death and Bereavement Across Cultures*, 2nd edn. Hove: Routledge, 23–41.

Saunders, C. (1998) Foreword. In: Doyle, D., Hanks, G. and MacDonald, N. (eds) *Oxford Textbook of Palliative Medicine*, 2nd edn. Oxford: Oxford University Press, v–ix.

Scholes, J. (2006) *Developing Expertise in Critical Care Nursing*. Chichester: Wiley/Blackwell.

Seymour, R.J., Payne, S., Reid, D., Sargeant, A., Skilbeck, J. and Smith, P. (2005) Ethical and methodological issues in palliative care studies. *Journal of Research in Nursing*, 10 (2): 169–188.

Shannon, S.E., Long-Sutehall, T. and Coombs, M. (2011) Conversations in end of life care: communication tools for critical care practitioners. *Nursing in Critical Care*, 16 (3): 124–129.

Simard, J. (2013) *The End of Life Namaste Care Program for People with Dementia*. Baltimore, MD: Health Professions Press.

Slapper, G. and Kelly, D. (2015) *The English Legal System 2015–2016*, 16th edn. London: Routledge.

Stacpoole, M., Hockley, J., Thompsell, A., Simard, J. and Volicer, L. (2014) The Namaste Care programme can reduce behavioural symptoms in care home residents with advanced dementia. *International Journal of Geriatric Psychiatry*, 30: 702–709.

Stayt, L.C. (2009) Death, empathy and self-preservation: the emotional labour of caring for families of the critically ill in adult intensive care. *Journal of Clinical Nursing*, 18: 1267–1275.

Stiefel, F., Nakamura, K., Terui, T. and Ishitani, K. (2017) Collusions between patients and clinicians in end-of-life care: why clarity matters. *Journal of Pain Symptom Management*. Available from: www.ncbi.nlm.nih.gov/pubmed/28062352 (accessed 12 January 2017).

Stroebe, M. and Schut, D. (1999) The dual process model of coping with bereavement: rationale and description. *Death Studies*, 23 (3): 197–224.

Suicide Act 1961 (c.60) (online). Available from: www.legislation.gov.uk/ukpga/Eliz2/ 9–10/60/data.pdf (accessed 1 September 2016).

Taheri, N. (2008) *Healthcare in Islamic History and Experience* (online). Available from: http://ethnomed.org/cross-cultural-health/religion/health-care-in-islamic-history-and-experience (accessed 15 November 2016).

Taylor, H. (2015) Legal and ethical issues in end of life care: implications for primary healthcare. *Primary Healthcare*, 25 (4): 32–40.

Thomas, C. (2008) Dying: places and preferences. In: Payne, S., Seymour, J. and Ingleton, C. (eds) *Palliative Care Nursing: Principles and Evidence Based Practice*, 2nd edn. Maidenhead: McGraw-Hill, Open University Press.

Thompson, D.R., Hamilton, D.K., Cadenhead, C.D. et al. (2012) Guidelines for intensive care unit design. *Critical Care Medicine*, 40 (5): 1586 (online). Available from: www.learnicu.org/SiteAssets/Pages/Guidelines/Guidelines%20for%20intensive%20care%20unit%20design.pdf (accessed 5 July 2013).

Tiberini, R. and Richardson, H. (2015) *Rehabilitative palliative care: enabling people to live fully until they die: a challenge for the 21st century*. London: Hospice UK.

(The) Times (2017) (online). Available from: www.thetimes.co.uk/article/brexit-blamed-for-soaring-assaults-on-hospital-staff-tbpwxg397 (accessed 3 April 2017).

Tingle, J. and Cribb, A. (2007) *Nursing Law and Ethics*, 3rd edn. Oxford: Blackwell.

Tschudin, V. (ed.) (2003) *Approaches to Ethics: Nursing Beyond Boundaries*. Boston: Harcourt.

Tuffrey-Wijne, I. and McEnhill, L. (2008) Communication difficulties and intellectual disability in end-of-life care. *International Journal of Palliative Nursing*, 14 (4): 189–194.

Twycross, R.G. (2003) *Introducing Palliative Care*, 4th edn. Oxford: Oxford University Press.

W (by her litigation friend B) v *M (by her litigation friend the Official Solicitor) and others* [2011] All Er 1313 (online). Available from: Lexis®Library (accessed 1 September 2016).

Walker, R. and Read, S. (2010) The Liverpool Care Pathway in intensive care: an exploratory study of doctor and nurse perceptions. *International Journal of Palliative Nursing*, 16 (6): 267–273.

Walsh, D. and Nelson, K. (2003) Communication of a cancer diagnosis: patients' perception of when they were first told they had cancer. *American Journal of Hospice and Palliative Care*, 20 (1): 52–56.

Wilson, M.H. (2008) 'There's just something about Ron': one nurse's healing presence amidst failing hearts. *Journal of Holistic Nursing*, 26 (4): 303–307.

Woodrow, P. (2011) *Intensive Care Nursing: A Framework for Practice*, 3rd edn. London: Routledge.

World Health Organization (1990) *Technical Report*, series 804. Geneva: World Health Organization.

World Health Organization (2012a) *WHO Definition of Palliative Care* (online). Available from: www.who.int/cancer/palliative/definition/en (accessed 16 March 2013).

World Health Organization (2012b) *Rehabilitation* (online). Available from: www.who.int/topics/rehabilitation/en/ (accessed 22 November 2016).

Zimmerman, C., Del Piccolo, L. and Mazzi, M.A. (2003) Patient cues and medical interviewing in general practice: examples of the application of sequential analysis. *Epidemiologia e Psichiatria Sociale*, 12 (2): 115–123.

Index